Mastering the ATI TEAS 7: Your Path to Success

Insider Strategies, Practice Tests, and Real-Life Insights for TEAS Mastery.

Introduction: Embarking on Your TEAS Journey

You must have heard that becoming a nurse really takes hard work. You must have also heard that the ATI TEAS (The Test of Essential Academic Skills) examination is one of the toughest, stressful, and overwhelming part of the application process. Right now, you may even be standing at the crossroads of excitement and uncertainty, feeling so scared and unsure of what to expect from the TEAS examination, how it works, what you need to do and if you can actually achieve them. Do not worry yourself to death.

Why? You can successfully scale through this. You are not alone in this journey. Infact! the uncertainties and fears are absolutely normal and there are many aspiring healthcare professionals standing where you stand now, looking at the Test of Essential Academic Skills (TEAS) as both a challenge and a ticket to their dreams.

The difference between you and them right now is that you've gotten a guide that will make your dream come true. With this guide, the ATI TEAS would no longer be daunting to you; as it will walk you through the process, from understanding the test format to studying the core material. In the chapters ahead, we'll walk hand in hand, demystifying the intricacies of the ATI TEAS examination. You'll also get a taste of what it's like to take the exam, with practice tests and quizzes that simulate the real thing.

So, here's to your dedication, your dreams, and the journey ahead. As you turn the pages of this guide, remember that every piece of knowledge gained and every practice question conquered is a stride closer to the nurse you're destined to become.

Chapter 1:

Understanding the TEAS - Format and Content

What is the ATI TEAS 7?

In simplest terms, the ATI TEAS 7 or Test of Essential Academic Skills is a standardized or entrance test that is used to measure the academic readiness of any one aspiring to get into the nursing school. You could liken it to the test you took before you were accepted into high school or college. The main goal of this test is to assess the skills and knowledge of aspiring nurses before being admitted into the nursing school; as well as to measure your ability to succeed in nursing school and as a nurse.

Why do you have to take the TEAS?

The ATI TEAS 7 is intended to assess your ability to think critically, apply any knowledge, and communicate effectively in any academic setting. It's not a test that assess you on nursing-specific knowledge or topics but rather, it's a test of your general knowledge and academic skills. The test is so important that it is administered by the Assessment Technologies Institute (ATI) and every nursing school in the United States and every existing field wants your TEAS 7 score to be included within your examination application. The test covers every subject an aspiring nursing student will be expected to know before and after getting into nursing school.

THE TEAS 7 SUBJECT SECTIONS, TEST FORMAT AND QUESTION TYPES.
What does the TEAS consist of?

Subject Areas/Sections:

More like the different chapters of a book, the TEAS 7 has four test sections: Reading, Mathematics, Science, and English and Language Usage.

> **The Reading Section:**

Knowing how to read the medical documents and communicate them effectively to the patient is a valuable asset that every aspiring nurse must possess hence, this section aims to evaluate your critical thinking skills and ability to extract relevant information from diverse contexts.

The section is broken into 3 different areas in addition to the pretest questions and the test candidates will be presented with passages for you to read and answer questions about the information presented. This is called comprehensive analysis.
Beyond mere comprehension, the focus is on finding main ideas of the passage, as well as drawing inferences, and interpreting the authors intent of writing. You will be required to answer questions related to the areas of:
 I.   Key Ideas and Details
 II. Craft and Structure, and
 III. Integration of Knowledge and Ideas.

→ **Key Ideas & Details**
This section quizzes you on the objective aspects of writing especially within the aspect of factual evidence and its uses. It also quizzes you about the structure of persuasive arguments. To accurately answer the 15 questions in this section, you need to know how to:
- Interpret events in a sequence
- Locate specific information in a text
- Summarize a multi-paragraph text
- Make inferences and draw conclusions about a text's meaning and purpose.
- Demonstrate comprehension of written directions.
- Analyze, interpret, and apply information from charts, graphs, and other visuals.

→ **Craft & Structure**
This category gathers its 9 questions on the stylistic aspects of writing. You need to know how to:
- Evaluate an author's point of view in a given text
- Evaluate an author's purpose in a given text
- Distinguish between fact and opinion
- Use context to interpret the meaning of words and phrases.

→ **Integration of Knowledge & Ideas**
This sub-sections specifically deals with research and evidence. To successfully answer all the 15 questions in this area, you will be asked to fulfill these tasks:
- Evaluate an argument

- Compare and contrast the themes expressed in one or more texts
- Use evidence from a text to make predictions and inferences and to draw conclusions
- Evaluate and integrate data from multiple sources across various formats.

➤ The Mathematics Section:

The Mathematics section of the TEAS exam requires you to showcase your quantitative reasoning skills as it comprises 2 sub-content areas in addition to the pretest questions. It seeks to assess your basic maths and problem-solving skills, as well as your ability to apply the mathematical calculations and measurements to real-world scenarios.

You will also be provided with a 4-function calculator used for solving various maths problems on the exam day.

As a test candidate, you will be expected to answer questions about:

   I.   Number and Algebra
  II.   Measurement and Data.

→ Numbers & Algebra

In this sub-section, you'll be asked questions on algebras and numbers. The 16 questions which you would need to answer features various types of numerical expressions ranging from ratios, rational numbers, proportions, estimations, and percentages. You will be asked to:

- Solve real-world problems involving percentages
- Convert among non-negative fractions, decimals, and percentages
- Solve real-world problems involving proportions
- Solve real-world problems involving ratios and rates of change
- Solve real-world situations using expressions, equations, and inequalities
- Compare and order rational numbers
- Solve equations with one variable
- Perform arithmetic operations with rational numbers
- Solve real-world problems using one- or multi-step operations with real numbers and
- Apply estimation strategies and rounding rules to real-world problems.

→ Measurement & Data

This sub-section features quantitative questions and figures. The 18 questions which would be asked in this section revovles around the various units of measurement, different types of data presentations, and several geometric and statistical properties and principles. Here's what you'll be asked to do:

- Calculate geometric quantities

- Explain the relationship between two variables
- Interpret relevant information from tables, charts, and graphs
- Evaluate the information in data sets, tables, charts, and graphs using statistics
- Convert with and between standard and metric systems.

➤ The Science Section:

Nursing and science work closely together. Infact, they cannot do without each other in the healthcare world. Most especially because medicine relies on science to find ways to help people with their health issues. As an aspiring nurse, you'll learn to use scientific methods to understand how the body functions.

For example, you'll be trained to read vital signs and know the signs of different illnesses in order to identify and diagnose health problems in your patients. This Science section of the TEAS exam is broken into 3 sub-sections and it does include the pretest questions. Here, you'll be required to answer specific questions in:

I. Human Anatomy
II. Physiology and Life
III. Physical Sciences
IV. Scientific Reasoning

→ Human Anatomy & Physiology

This sub-section quizzes on the biological processes of the human body and how the different body systems function both separately and together. You need to learn about **the description of the anatomy and physiology of the following systems:**

- Male and female reproductive systems
- Integumentary system
- Endocrine system
- Urinary system
- Immune system
- Skeletal system
- Cardiovascular system
- Digestive system
- Nervous system
- Muscular system
- Respiratory system and
- The general orientation of the human anatomy

→ Biology

The 9 questions asked in this sub-section deals with the various aspects of cell structure, microorganisms, and protein structure. Here's what you would be asked to do:

- Describe the role of microorganisms in disease
- Describe cell structure, function, and organization
- Describe the structure and function of the basic macromolecules in a biological system
- Describe the relationship between genetic material and the structure of proteins and
- Apply concepts underlying Mendel's laws of inheritance.

→ Chemistry

The 8 questions asked in this sub-section hinges on the various aspects of chemical reactions, acids and bases, atomic structure, and properties of matter. You should study on:

- How to recognize basic atomic structure
- Know the physical properties and changes of matter
- Describe chemical reactions
- Demonstrate how conditions affect chemical reactions
- Understand properties of solutions
- Describe concepts of acids and bases.

→ Scientific Reasoning

The 9 questions asked in this sub-section deal with your knowledge of science on a basic level. No hard things. Hence you should learn properly on how to:

- Predict relationships among events, objects, and processes
- Apply the scientific method to interpret a scientific investigation
- Use basic scientific measurements and tools
- Apply logic and evidence to a scientific explanation.

Your questions will majorly revolve around the core concepts of human anatomy and physiology, chemistry, scientific reasoning, and biology. Hence, it is important that you study these areas properly because the essence of the TEAS exam is hinged on these areas. Which is to gauge the candidates' readiness to enter any health science-related program or school.

It is also important to ensure that you do not focus on memorization alone but on understanding the fundamental scientific principles when reading for this section because the test questions will test your ability to think critically about any scientific information.

➤ The English and Language Usage Section:

You might wonder why this is part of a nursing exam. Well, as a nurse, you'll be talking to many patients, colleagues, and supervisors every day and to communicate well, you'll need to be grounded on the basics of English, like how to write and express your thoughts clearly. This skill helps you respond to different situations as a nurse and choose your words wisely. Also, during your nursing education, you'll most likely be assigned to write essays and reports. Therefore, being able to express your ideas is crucial for success and graduation.

This final section of the TEAS exam scrutinizes your language proficiency. It's all about how well you use and communicate in English. This section also contains 3 sub-areas including the pretest questions and it is a bit similar to the TEAS reading section, however you will need an advanced understanding of the English language. Here, you'll be required to answer specific questions on:

I.   Conventions of Standard English
II.   Knowledge of the English Language
III. Use of Language and Vocabulary For Expressing Ideas in Writing.

To get every mark in this test section, you should focus on:

→ Conventions of Standard English

All 12 questions asked in this sub-section is hinged on the basic knowledge, skills, and abilities you have relating to the conventions of standard English. This is what you'll be asked to do:

- Use correct sentence structures
- Use conventions of standard English spelling
- Use conventions of standard English pronunciation

→ Knowledge of Language

All 11 questions in this sub-section is created to evaluate your understanding of how language can be utilized when writing. Here's what you should read on:

- How to use grammar to enhance clarity in writing
- How to develop a well-organized paragraph
- How to find out if a language meets the needs of a particular audience

→ Use of Language and Vocabulary For Expressing Ideas in Writing.

All 10 questions asked in this sub-section is meant to test how you're able to effectively communicate your ideas when writing through the use of an advanced level vocabulary and grammar. You need to make indepth study on:

- How to apply basic knowledge of the elements of the writing process to communicate effectively
- How to determine the meanings of words by analyzing word parts.

All these questions are asked to ensure that you communicate ideas clearly and precisely as an aspiring healthcare professional. This subject is also the shortest section of the TEAS 7 examination. Both in the number of questions asked (37 questions) and the time allotted to the questions (37 minutes). Also, in each subject area, you will be required to answer some pretest questions and questions pertaining to several different areas. As you read on, we will discuss in detail the number of questions in each section.

How does The TEAS 7 Test Questions look like?

If you've read to this point, it's certain that you have been wondering about the exam questions format and if the TEAS 7 test is a multiple choice question format. Well, the answer is Yes! The test is indeed in a multiple choice format however, Multiple-choice questions are not the only type of questions asked during the TEAS examination.

Previously in the TEAS 6, only multiple-choice questions were the type of questions given to the test candidate. But the TEAS 7 changed the whole system as this new computerized version of the TEAS test comprises of four new question types in addition to multiple-choice. They are:

- **Multiple-Choice:**

This type of question requires you to choose one correct answer from four options provided. Some questions may not be only text but may include charts, exhibits, or graphics.

> **Simplify the following expression:**
>
> $7+16-(5+6\times3)-10\times2$
>
> A. -42
> B. -20
> C. 23
> D. 20

- **Multiple-Select**

This type of question requires you to choose all correct answers from four or more options. This means that there may be more than one correct answer. For this type of question, a prompt will appear to you asking that you "select all that apply." So, you need to select all the right answers to get the question correct else, the selection of any incorrect answer will make the question be marked as incorrect with no score point given.

> **Which of the following transitional words or phrases can be used to indicate contrast? (Select all that apply**.)
>
> A. Regardless
> B. Furthermore
> C. On the other hand
> D. Moreover

- **Supply Answer**

This type of question do not provide any answer option. Rather, the question demands that you "fill in the blank" or to provide an answer to the question asked. Here, numbers and words are acceptable as correct answers.

> **Complete the sentence:**
>
> Jane has $40, and each case of cola costs $3.50, so she can buy a total of .... cases of cola.

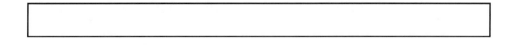

- **Hot Spot**

This type of question gives you an image that contains two to five clickable areas. You are expected to click on the correct area of the image that answers the question.

> Select the hot spot that contains the correct answer.
>
> Maria is numbering the points of a pentagon from 1 to 5. She labels the top point as point 1 and continues anti-clockwise. Which of the following would Mariah label as point 3?
>
>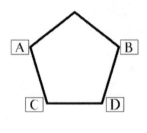

- **Ordered Response**

This type of question requires you to correctly arrange responses in the correct order by dragging them. Each question gives you four to six responses, and you must drag each option from a box on the left to a box on the right. If you drag any answer in the wrong order, the whole question is marked incorrect with no score given.

Arrange the following fractions in ascending order:	Arrange Here:
1. ⅓	
2. ⅖	
3. ⅜	
4. 5/12	

How many Questions are on the TEAS Test?

To answer this question, you need to know how many questions the TEAS test contain as well as understand the TEAS test breakdown and the total number of questions for each section.

The TEAS test contains 170 questions in total with 45 questions in the Reading section for 55 minutes, 38 questions in the Mathematics section for 57 minutes, 50 questions in the Science section 60 minutes, and 37 questions in the English and Language Usage section for 37 minutes. All these question is expected to be answered within the time alloted, which is 209 minutes in total or 3.5 hours, with an extra 10-minute break after the Mathematics test section.

It is important to also be aware that your score will only be affected by 150 of these questions as the other 20 sample questions also known as pretest questions will evaluate you differently and they do not add any points to your score. These pretest questions with no score serve as questions that may potentially appear on future releases of the exam and they are meant to either gauge which questions should be included to the TEAS 7 future test, which could be too challenging or unfit for the test.

- Tip: When you are done clicking your answers, ensure you review your answers before submitting your exam.

The table below shows what the TEAS test consists of and the TEAS exam breakdown for each section.

SUBJECT AREAS AND SUB-SECTIONS	NUMBER OF QUESTIONS AND TIME ALLOTED
The Reading Section:	45 QUESTIONS • 55 Mins
Key Ideas & Details	15
Craft & Structure	9
Integration of Knowledge & Ideas	15
Pretest Questions	6
The Mathematics Section:	38 QUESTIONS • 57 Mins
Numbers & Algebra	18
Measurement & Data	6
Pretest Questions	4
The Science Section:	50 QUESTIONS • 60 Mins
Human Anatomy & Physiology	18
Biology	9
Chemistry	8
Scientific Reasoning	9
Pretest Questions	6

The English and Language Usage Section:	37 QUESTIONS • 37 Mins
Conventions of Standard English	12
Knowledge of Language	11
Use of Language and Vocabulary For Expressing Ideas in Writing	10
Pretest Questions	4

7 Essential Strategies to Help You Master the Test Format and Succeed
Strategies for Familiarization with the Test Format

Preparing for your TEAS 7 exam demands more than just studying your subjects. It demands that you familiarize yourself the test format and master them. It is very important that you do this because understanding the test format gives you a roadmap for what to expect during the test.

When you know how the test is organized and the types of questions you'll face, you will feel more confident, less anxious, comfortable and less stressed. Plus, mastering the format helps you develop smart study strategies tailored to the specific demands of the test, making you focus on the areas where you need the most help. In short, familiarizing yourself with the test format is essential for effective preparation and success of your TEAS 7 exam.

Here are some key strategies to help you become acquainted with the format:

➢ **Utilize Official Study Materials:**

One of the most effective ways to get ready for the TEAS test is by using the official study materials from ATI. These materials, including the official TEAS study guide are meticulously designed to give you a good understanding of what the exam the structure and content is like.

The official study guide is like your main tool for getting ready. It gives you detailed information about the test format, the kinds of questions you'll see, and what subject areas are covered. It also has sample practice questions accompanied by thorough explanations that will make you understand why certain answers are right and the common mistakes to avoid.

14

By using these official study materials, you will gain a solid foundation of knowledge and mastery with the intricacies of the TEAS 7 exam. You'll become accustomed to the types of questions you'll encounter, the level of difficulty, and the overall expectations for each section of the test. Moreover, the official study materials are created by the same organization responsible for administering the TEAS exam, and you know they are accurate, reliable, and relevant to the actual test experience.

You can trust that they'll give you a good idea of what to expect on test day. Also, using these materials as part of your study plan helps you stay organized and focused. You can use them to figure out what to study, where you need to improve, and you're progress as you get ready. You'll also know that you've put in the work and have what you need to tackle all challenges and do your best.

> ## ➤ Engage in Practice Tests:

Practice tests are invaluable tools for the real TEAS exam. They help you get used to how the test works and also hone your TEAS 7 test-taking skills. These tests are actually designed to replicate the actual TEAS exam, so they give you a good idea of what to expect when you take the real test.

When you often engage in taking the practice tests, you can get used to how fast you need to go (pacing), the questions structure, and the different types of questions you'll see on the exam day. These practice tests give you the opportunity to experience the time constraints of each section and helps you learn how to manage your time better during the actual exam whilst making sure you can answer all the questions in each section.

Practice tests also allows you to assess your strengths and weaknesses across different subject areas. It reveals what you're good at and what you need to work on. By looking at your results after self- assessment, you can identify which areas you need to study more and which areas you're already doing well in. Furthermore, practice tests provide valuable opportunities for you to become accustomed to the format and style of questions asked on the TEAS exam.

Whether it's multiple-choice, fill-in-the-blank, or scenario-based questions, you can gain mastery of the different question types and come up with strategies for answering them. And don't forget, doing practice tests prepares you mentally for the actual exam as it builds your ability to perform well under pressure and increases your confidence. Remember, you must never skip this crucial part in preparation for your TEAS 7 examination.

Here are examples of practice test questions which you might encounter for each section of the TEAS exam:

 Sample Question:

1. Reading Section:
   Read the following passage:

"The Industrial Revolution marked a significant shift in human history, bringing about unprecedented technological advancements and societal transformations. From the mechanization of production processes to the rise of urbanization, the impacts of this period are still felt today. In what ways did the Industrial Revolution shape modern society?"

Based on the passage, which of the following statements best summarizes the main idea?
   A) The Industrial Revolution led to technological advancements and societal changes that continue to influence modern society.
   B) The Industrial Revolution was a period of great unrest and conflict, with little long-term impact on society.
   C) The Industrial Revolution primarily affected rural communities, leading to a decline in agricultural practices.
   D) The Industrial Revolution had minimal impact on societal structures and technological development.

2. Mathematics Section:

   Solve the following equation for x:
   $2x + 5 = 15$
   A) $x = 5$
   B) $x = 10$
   C) $x = 15$
   D) $x = 20$

3. Science Section:

The human circulatory system consists of which of the following components?
   A) Heart, lungs, liver
   B) Brain, spinal cord, nerves

C) Heart, blood vessels, blood

D) Kidneys, bladder, ureters

4. English and Language Usage Section:

<u>Choose the sentence that is grammatically correct:</u>

A) The cat sat on it's mat.

B) The cat sat on its mat.

C) The cat sat on it is mat.

D) The cat sat on it mat.

➤ Review Your Practice Test Results:

After completing the practice tests, it is important to look closely at the results and identify your areas of strength and areas that need improvement. Doing this will push you into developing better study plans and you'll focus on areas that will have the greatest impact on your overall test performance.

One way to review your practice test results is to look at each question and the answer you chose. If you got a question right, think about why you chose that answer and make sure you understand the concept. If you got a question wrong or weren't sure of the answer, read the explanations provided and see where you went wrong.

Also, pay attention to your performance in different subject areas of the test. Are there subjects, topics, or types of questions where you always struggle and fail? Are there subject areas where you perform better than expected? Knowing these patterns guides you into developing study strategies that are tailored to improve your weak areas. Are there sections where time was insufficient to complete all questions?

In addition to this, think about how long it took you to finish each section of the practice test too. Are there sections where you spent too much time? Did you run out of time on others? Time management is very important when it comes to the real TEAS exam, so practice pacing yourself effectively to ensure you can complete each section within the allotted time.

Lastly, keep track of your improvement over time and adjust your study plans when needed. You should also look back at old practice tests and compare your previous and recent results as it will gauge your readiness for the exam. In short, reviewing practice test results is a big part of your getting ready for the TEAS exam because by carefully reviewing your performance, identifying subjects or topics that should be worked on, and making better study plans, you can do your best on test day.

➢ Understand the Question Types:

It's important to know the different types of questions you'll see on the TEAS test because each section has its own kinds of questions, and knowing them gives you precision and increases your readiness for the test.

In the Reading section, you will encounter a variety of question types designed to assess your reading comprehension skills. They may include Identification of the main idea in a passage, discerning what the author is trying to say (inference), writing the contextual meaning of words, and the author's purpose. By understanding the different question types, you can learn how to find the answers in the reading passages. as soon as possible.

Similarly, in the Mathematics section, you will encounter questions on arithmetic, algebra, geometry, and data interpretation. The most common question formats used in this section are multiple-choice questions, word problems, and quantitative comparisons are common question formats in this section. Candidates should familiarize themselves with the specific skills and concepts tested in each question type to ensure readiness on test day. Mastering these kinds of questions gives you an advantage on the exam day.

The Science section of the TEAS exam assesses you on your understanding of core scientific concepts in anatomy, physiology, chemistry, and biology. You'll see questions about reading data(data interpretation), concept application, experimental design, and understanding scientific ideas and their application to solving real problems, and. Focusing on these question types helps you focus your study efforts.

Finally, In the English and Language Usage section, you will encounter questions focusing on on grammar, punctuation, sentence structure, and language usage. Some questions ask you to fill in the missing word, identify errors in a sentence or revise a passage hence, familiarizing yourself with these types of questions will help you brush up on your English skills and achieve your desired scores in the TEAS 7 test.

➢ Practice Time Management:

Managing your time well during the TEAS exam is super important and if want to make sure you have enough time to answer all the questions without feeling rushed, you'll need to try this time management tips.

First, try timing yourself when you take practice tests. Setting a timer for each section to mimic the real test's time limits will help you get used to how long you have left for each question and section. Next, pay attention to how much time you spend on each question. If you find yourself taking too long on a question, make a note to come back to it later. Don't get stuck – move on to the next question and come back if you have time.

It's also helpful to draft a plan for how you'll spend your time during the exam. For example, you might decide to spend a certain amount of time on each section, or you might prioritize certain types of questions. Just ensure you experiment with different strategies to see what works best for you before the exam.

Finally, work on answering questions efficiently without sacrificing accuracy. Learn to recognize when to skip a question and come back to it later, rather than getting stuck and wasting time. You should also practice how to make educated guesses and move on to the next question when necessary. By practicing these time management tips, you'll be able to tackle each section of the exam with ease, knowing you have a plan in place to manage your time effectively.

> **Utilize Additional Resources:**

In addition to the official study materials and practice tests, there are many other resources available you can use in preparation for your TEAS 7 exam. These extra tools can give you more practice examples and explainations as well as offer useful tips to help you understand the test better. They include:

- **Review Books:** Consider checking out review books made specifically for the TEAS 7 exam. These books often cover all the important topics, include practice questions, and make detailed explanations that will reinforce what you have studied.

- **Online Tutorials:** This is another advantageous option. You can find lots of videos and lectures online that go over TEAS exam topics. Some of them are free on the websites while others may demand you pay a small token for it. Either way, they can be really helpful for getting a better grasp of the any subject or topic.

- **Flashcards:** Flashcards are another handy tool for studying key concepts and terms. You can create your own or use ones that are already made sets available online or in study guides. They're easy to review anytime, anywhere, and they help you remember important information.

- **Study Groups:** It is very important to join or form study groups with classmates or friends who are also preparing for the TEAS exam. Studying with others allows you to share resources, discuss challenging topics, and quiz each other in different topics and subjects. It is also a fun way to learn together and to remain motivated to study.

- **Online Forums:** Online forums are also a good place to get support, strategies and learn more. There are lots of forums and discussion groups where people talk about TEAS exam preparation and these forums provide you with opportunities to ask questions, share study tips, and connect with other candidates preparing for the exam.

- **Educational Websites:** Check out educational websites that offer interactive quizzes, practice exercises, and study guides tailored to the TEAS exam subjects. These websites often provide you targeted practice in different subjects and give you instant feedback on your progress. Finally, by using these additional resources alongside your main study materials, you can boost your preparation for the TEAS exam. Also try out different resources to see what works best for your learning style and schedule.

➤ Seek Feedback and Support:

Seeking feedback and support is essential during your preparation for the TEAS exam. Let me explain why it's so important and how it can help you succeed. Imagine you're studying hard for the TEAS exam, but you're feeling a bit unsure and stuck on certain topics. Maybe you're not sure if you're studying the right things, or you're struggling to understand some concepts. This is where seeking feedback and support can really make a big difference.

Firstly, don't hesitate to ask your teachers, tutors, friends, or classmates for help. They've been through the exam process before you and can offer valuable advice and guidance. Whether it's clarifying a confusing concept, explaining a tricky problem, or providing study tips, getting feedback from others can help you overcome challenges and improve your understanding.

This is why joining or forming a study group with classmates can also be incredibly helpful. Studying with others allows you to share resources, discuss difficult topics, and quiz each other. It's a great way to learn from each other's experiences and support one another through the ups and downs of exam preparation.

In addition to this, participating in online forums and discussion groups dedicated to TEAS exam preparation can provide a sense of community and belonging. You can connect with fellow test-takers, ask questions, share study strategies, and offer encouragement.

Knowing that others are going through the same process can be reassuring and motivating so, it is important that you understand that seeking feedback and support isn't just about getting answers to specific questions but about building confidence and resilience. When you reach out to others for help, you're showing that you are committed to success and willing to do whatever it takes to achieve your goals.

Always remember, you don't have to go through the TEAS exam preparation process alone. There are people who want to see you succeed and who are willing to support you every step of the way. So don't be afraid to ask for help, seek feedback, and lean on others for support – it can make all the difference in your TEAS exam preparation journey.

Personal Insight
How Understanding the Test Format Transformed My Experience: Emily's Personal TEAS Exam Story.

Let me share a personal story to illustrate how effective understanding the TEAS test format is to you.

Meet Emily, my best friend. She's a determined student with aspirations of pursuing a career in nursing. Like many aspiring healthcare professionals, she faced the daunting challenge of preparing for the TEAS exam. Emily had heard stories of its difficulty and knew that success on this exam was crucial for gaining admission to nursing school.

As she began her preparing for her TEAS exam she quickly realized that understanding the test format was key to her success so she spent countless hours studying her subjects. However, my best friend still felt a sense of unease about what to expect on test day.
But everything changed one day when she bumped into a TEAS practice website while making research about the TEAS test. So she decided to take a practice test under timed conditions to simulate the real exam environment. As she worked through each section, she paid close attention to the format of the questions and how they were structured.

At first, Emily confessed to me that she felt overwhelmed by the time alloted to her and the sheer volume of questions to answer. But as she continued, she began to notice patterns in the types of questions asked and the strategies needed to approach them effectively. After two days of consistent practice, she realized that by understanding the format of the test, she could approach each question with more confidence and efficiency.

On the fourth day, she clicked the review button on the website to review her practice test results on the website and was amazed at how much her understanding of the test questions and format had improved. She immediately flew to our Buddy couch to map out other areas where she still struggled and drafted out a plan to focus her study efforts on those specific topics. Armed with this newfound insight, my friend explained to me whenever we met in church that she felt more prepared and confident to tackle the TEAS exam head-on.

On the test day, Emily said to me that she walked into the testing center confidently and when she sat down for the test, she approached each question methodically, drawing from the strategies she had learned during her two months preparation. When my friend finally received her scores, she was so thrilled to see that her hard work had paid off that she ran over to my house with her hair bonnet on because, she achieved a score that surpassed her expectations and imaginations. Smiles. Now my Emily's dream of becoming a nurse is already a reality.

I really think you should do this too. What do you think?

Chapter 2:

Time Management Mastery

Time is a precious resource. It is something we can't see or touch, but shapes every aspect of our lives. From the very moment you wake up to the last minute you get to lay on your bed with your eyes closed, time ticks away. And when it comes to writing your ATI TEAS 7 exam, time management becomes even more critical.

You should think of time management as your secret weapon in the battle against the ticking clock during your TEAS examination. It's like a magic wand that will help you navigate through the test with just an easy wave and confidence. Without proper time management skills, you could find yourself scrambling to finish questions on the exam day. You'll feel stressed, unhappy, burnt out, tensed and also risk not completing the exam on time.

So why is time management so important for the TEAS exam?

Well, also imagine this: You have a limited amount of time to answer a bunch of questions covering various subjects like math, science, English, and reading comprehension. Each question is like a puzzle piece, and you need to fit them all together within the given time frame. You know, if you do not manage your time wisely in a situation as this, you will end up leaving some pieces behind and not completing the puzzle – or in this case, the exam.

But fear not! This is why this chapter was written for you! In this chapter, we'll give you time management practice techniques that will simulate the exam, help you walk confidently into your TEAS 7 exam environment and conquer it! We'll start by making you understand the time constraints of each section of the exam and why it's essential to be aware of them. Then, we'll explore effective time management strategies that will help you pace yourself, prioritize questions, stay calm under pressure and maintain focused throughout the exam. All this is to enable you perform at your best on the exam day!

How To Effectively Manage Your Time And Complete Each Section Of Your TEAS 7 Exam Within The Alloted Time
(Time Management Strategies for the TEAS Exam)

When it comes to conquering the TEAS exam, effective time management is your best friend. Here are some simple yet powerful strategies that'll help you make the most of your time:

➢ Prioritize Your Questions:

Just like in real life, not all questions on the TEAS exam are created equal. Some are quick, straightforward, and easy to answer, while others would require more time, effort, and thought to answer. To maximize your efficiency, you need to start by scanning through the questions and identifying those that you feel most confident answering. Tackle them first. Answering these questions first will help you build momentum, gain more marks, and save time for the more challenging and tougher questions ones later on.

➢ Allocate Time Wisely:

Once you've prioritized your questions, by picking those which you're more familiar with, it's essential to allocate your time wisely. In the first chapter, we've explained the total time available for each section and sub-section. Each section of the TEAS exam has a designated time limit, so you'll need to divide the total number of minutes for that section by the number of questions to determine how much time you can afford to spend on each. You can do this during your practice test to become more familiar with your timing and how fast you answer a question from any section and sub-section. This strategic approach ensures that you pace your self and distribute your time wisely without spending too much time on any single question.

➢ Use the Mark and Review Feature:

This strategy is very useful when you encounter a tricky or challenging question that stumps you or requires more time to answer. Rather than dwelling on that particular question for too long, simply use the mark and review feature to flag the question and move on to the next question. This technique allows you to keep moving forward without getting stuck and losing precious time, knowing that you can come back to a question later if the time allocated for that section hasn't ended.

➢ Break It Down:

Sometimes, the sheer size of the TEAS 7 exam questions can feel overwhelming but remember, you don't have to tackle it all at once. Break down the questions into smaller, manageable chunks to make it more approachable and easier to tackle. When preparing for the test and while you're taking the TEAS examination, you could set mini-goals for yourself such as completing a certain number of questions within a specific time frame and celebrate your progress as you finish them.

➤ **Practice Time Management Techniques:**

Like any skill, effective time management takes practice. You need to familiarize yourself with time-saving techniques that would help you answer the different question types as soon as possible. For example, for multiple-choice questions, you could try eliminating obviously incorrect options instantly to narrow down your answer choices and to increase your chances of selecting the right answer quickly. You could also utilize shortcuts for your mathematical calculations.

Most importantly, ensure you incorporate timed practice tests into your study routine to simulate the real exam experience. This will help you become more comfortable with pacing yourself and allocating your time wisely, as well as reducing stress induced by the test on exam day. They will also help you increase your problem solving process and get you accustomed to working within the TEAS 7 time constraints.

With these time management strategies and techniques, you'll be better prepared to tackle the TEAS 7 exam with confidence and ease. Remember, practice makes perfect, so do not be afraid to experiment the different techniques to find what works best for you. So take a deep breath, keep calm, and manage your time like a pro. You've got this!

(Action Steps)
10 Practical Exercises
For Improving Time Management Skills

The pressure of completing each section of the TEAS 7 test within the time alloted to you makes developing a sturdy time management skills compulsive, especially if you want to attain your desired score. Here are 10 practical exercises designed to help you improve your time management skills as a TEAS 7 test candidate:

➤ **Set Specific Study Goals:**

Begin by setting clear and achievable study goals for your TEAS 7 exam preparation. Next, you need to break down larger study objectives into smaller, manageable tasks, and establish deadlines to keep yourself accountable. Or better still you can get an accountability partner. Someone to hold you by your word and study goals. By setting these specific goals, you can focus your study efforts more effectively and track your progress over time.

➤ **Create a Study Schedule:**

Passing the TEAS 7 exam requires you to develop a study schedule that outlines the topics and study times that you'll dedicatedly cover each day. You can use either a print or digital planner or calendar to organize your study schedule and ensure that you allocate sufficient time for each subject area which you'll be tested with on the TEAS 7 exam. Sticking to your study schedule consistently will make you gain steady progress towards your exam goals.

➤ **Prioritize Study Topics:**

Identify the most important and challenging topics on the TEAS 7 exam, and direct more study efforts to those areas. You should also direct your focus towards mastering difficult concepts and subject areas that you are less familiar with, while also reviewing and reinforcing your understanding of topics you are already comfortable with. Doing this will help you allocate your study time more effectively and focus on areas that will have the greatest impact on your overall performance.

➤ **Break Study Sessions into Manageable Segments:**

Breaking down your study sessions into smaller, more manageable segments will help you prevent burnout and maintain your focus for a longer study period. So, rather than trying to study for long periods without breaks, divide your study time into shorter intervals, with brief breaks in between for rest. This strategy will help you stay engaged and productive throughout your study sessions. It will also keep you from feeling easily overwhelmed or tired when you practice it.

➢ Use Active Learning Techniques:

Incorporating active learning techniques into your study routine will enhance your ability to comprehend and retain the information you've studied so far. So instead of passively reading or highlighting study materials, ensure you actively engage with the content by summarizing the key concepts in your own words, creating flashcards, or teaching the material to someone else. Doing this will deepen your understanding of the subject areas and topics.

➢ Practice Time Blocking:

In time blocking, all you need to do is to allocate dedicated blocks of time for studying each subject area tested on the TEAS 7 exam. With this, you can schedule focused study sessions for specific topics or subject areas, and also avoid multitasking or switching between subjects during each study session. You'll need to maintain concentration and make more efficient use of your study time if you truly want to pass your exam and become a healthcare professional.

➢ Set Time Limits for Practice Questions:

Challenging yourself to complete practice questions within specific time limits to simulate the timing constraints of the exam will make finishing your TEAS 7 exam feasible. It won't be a dream or desire but your reality. One you'll be so pleased to live in daily. All you need to do is to use a timer or stopwatch to track your progress and set time limits for each practice question or set of questions. This exercise will help you develop pacing strategies and also improve your ability to manage your time effectively during the actual examination.

➢ Review and Reflect on Your Study Sessions:

After you're done studying, set out time at the end of each study session to review your progress and reflect on your study habits and strategies. Evaluate which study techniques were most effective for you, and identify the areas where you struggled or encountered difficulties. By doing this, you will gain insights into your study strengths and weaknesses and also make the appropriate adjustments to your study approach.

➢ Practice Self-Discipline and Consistency:

This may sound so simple that you'll want to skip it but don't do that! You need this to pass your TEAS 7 exam and become a nurse. To develop self-discipline and consistency in your study habits, you only need to maintain a regular study routine. Study when you should and perform other activities when you should too. It's that easy. Set aside dedicated study times each day and commit to sticking to your study schedule, even when faced with distractions or competing priorities and your dream to become a healthcare professional is one step to becoming a reality.

➢ Reward Yourself for Milestones and Achievements:

Finally, do not forget to celebrate your progress and achievements along the way by rewarding yourself for reaching your study milestones, completing practice test in a short time or achieving challenging tasks. Set small rewards for yourself, such as taking a short break, enjoying your favorite snack, or engaging in a relaxing activity, after reaching your study goals or completing study sessions. This reward will keep you motivated and make you maintain a positive attitude towards your TEAS 7 exam preparation.

This is the end. However, ensure that you always approach your study sessions with focus, determination, and a positive mindset, and trust in your ability to succeed with diligent effort and practice. Do not look down on your self, abilities and dreams. Also give your self chances to improve. You can fail in one chance but not with many chances. These effective time management skills which you've read so far will make achieving your goals on the TEAS 7 exam attainable, So practice it!

Chapter 3:

Excelling in Reading Comprehension

When we talk about reading comprehension, we are referring to your ability to understand, interpret, and analyze written texts. So, it's not just about reading the words in a book or passage but understanding the meaning behind them. Reading comprehension, in its essence, is not just about reading words on a page; rather, it is about extracting meaning, identifying key information, and making connections between ideas presented in a passage.

This skill is super useful in understanding your TEAS 7 academic subjects and examination questions, in nursing school, and also in professional settings where complex documents, textbooks, research articles, journals, reports, patient charts, scenarios, and stories are commonly used to provide quality care and make informed decisions.

Now, why is reading comprehension so crucial, especially in the context of the TEAS 7 exam?

Well, let's start by considering the nature of the exam itself. The TEAS 7 exam assesses your readiness for entry into any nursing and allied health programs, which require strong academic skills, especially great reading comprehension. Also, in the examination, you will will encounter passages that cover a range of topics relevant to healthcare and the sciences.

These passages may include excerpts from textbooks, medical journals, research articles, and patient scenarios. Hence, to succeed in this exam, you must be able to comprehend these passages, extract key information, and apply it to answer questions accurately.

In this chapter, we'll focus on strategies that will improve your reading comprehension skills especially for the TEAS 7 exam. You'll learn reading techniques that will help you understand complex passages quickly, find the main ideas, and pick out the important details needed to answer the questions. Now let's cut the chase and get to the cheese!

7 Effective Reading Techniques That Will Help You Understand Complex TEAS 7 Passages Quickly And Easily

It's time to reveal to you the 7 techniques that will help you uncover the secrets hidden within any TEAS 7 comprehension passage or text. They are as follows:

➤ Active Reading

Active reading is like having a conversation with the text! It involves engaging with the text in a dynamic and purposeful manner. In active reading, you do not passively read or skim through the passage in a hurry, instead as a reader, you interact with the material by asking questions, making connections, and summarizing key points as you progress reading through the passage.

This reading technique increases your understanding of the passage deeper and helps you retain and recall more information from the passage. For example, imagine you are reading a passage from a TEAS 7 test prep book that discusses about the human circulatory system.

As an active reader, you engage with the text by:

- **Asking Questions:**

First off, as you read, question everything. Ask yourself questions as you read. Like, "What's the main job of the circulatory system?", "What role does capillaries play in the circulatory system?", or "How do arteries and veins differ?" You could also ask yourself what the main idea of the passage is and what evidence supports it. By asking questions, you're actively seeking answers and gaining a deeper, and better understanding of the material.

- **Making Predictions:**

Next, put on your fortune teller hat and try making predictions. Predict what is coming next based on the information you've gathered so far. For example, what do you think will happen? What is the effect of an action? Making predictions is essential because it will keep you engaged and help you anticipate the direction of the text.

- **Summarizing Key Points:**

Now, after reading a paragraph or section, summarize what you've read in your own words. Break down the main ideas and supporting details in a way you can easily remember and understand. The easiest way to do this is to imagine that you're telling a friend about the most interesting and captivating thing you learned from that passage. Summarizing your passages helps solidify your understanding and retention of the material.

- **Making Connections:**

Making connections involves relating the information in the passage to a personal experience or something you already know about. For example, if the passage discusses the role of blood vessels in transporting nutrients and oxygen, the reader might relate this to their knowledge of how a delivery system operates in a city. Building these bridges with connections makes the material more relatable, easier to understand and recall afterwards.

Next on, let do a simple run off of what you have read so far and apply it to a passage from the TEAS 7 exam on the human digestive system.

→ You'll ask questions like, "What organs are involved in digestion?" and "How does the digestive process work?"

→ You make predictions about what might come next in the passage based on what you already know about digestion.

→ After each section, you summarize the main points, like the role of enzymes in breaking down food.

→ And you connect the information to your own experiences, like remembering a time when you felt hungry and understanding how your body processed the food you ate.

By actively reading like this, you're not just skimming over the words—you're really digging into the material and getting the most out of your study time.

➤ Skimming

Skimming is like gliding over the surface of a text, picking up the main ideas without getting bogged down in the details. When you skim through a passage, you quickly glance through the passage to get an overview of the passage to identify it's main ideas and themes.

This reading technique allows you to grasp the overall structure and content of the passage without spending so much time reading every word and line in the text. This is also a valuable skill for quickly getting the gist of a passage, especially when you're racing against time in examinations like the TEAS 7.

You can skim through any passage effectively by:

- **Focusing on Headings and Subheadings:**

The headlines and subheadings will always give you a roadmap of the passage and highlight the main topics. So ensure you pay attention to them as you skim to get an overview of what the passage is about.

- **Reading the First and Last Sentences of Paragraphs:**

The first sentence often introduces the main idea, while the last sentence may provide a summary or conclusion. Diving off to read these important sentences will enable you grasp the key points without delving into every detail of the passage.

- **Looking for Keywords and Phrases:**

Look at for words or phrases that stand out, like names, dates, or terms related to the topic and underline or mark them. These keywords and phrases can give you clues about the main ideas and important information in the passage.

- **Paying Attention to Visual Aids:**

Always take note of tables, graphs, and images included in the passage as they can convey information to you quickly and succinctly. So, take a moment to glance at them when you find them, to see if they reinforce or clarify the main points in the text.

Now, here is a simple run off on what you have read so far in terms of applying skimming to a passage from the TEAS 7 exam. For example, if you're given a comprehension passage about the history of nursing, you'll skim through it by:

→ Quickly reading through the headings and subheadings to see what topics are covered, like "Early Origins of Nursing" or "Modern Nursing Practices."
→ You'll read the first and last sentences of each paragraph to get a sense of the main ideas, like learning about Florence Nightingale's contributions or the role of technology in modern nursing.
→ You'll look for keywords and phrases that stand out, such as "pioneering nurses" or "advancements in healthcare."
→ And you will pay attention to any visual aids, like a timeline or chart, that provide additional context or support the main ideas in the text.

If you skim this way, you can quickly grasp the main ideas of the passage during your TEAS 7 examination.

➢ Scanning

Scanning is like using a magnifying glass to quickly pinpoint specific information within a text. Or you could say it's like using a fast-forward button to find specific details in a text without reading every word. It deals with searching the passage. With scanning, you can locate key details or answers to specific questions quickly without having to read through the entire passage.

To scan effectively, you should:

- **Know What You're Looking For:**

Before you start scanning, you need to have a clear idea of what you're looking for. Whether it's a particular fact, term, answer to a question, or piece of data, knowing your target information will help you focus your search.

- **Look for Visual Cues:**

When scanning through a passage, it is important you quickly look for headings, subheadings, and the keywords that will guide your search.
These visual cues will give you hints on where to find the relevant information or answer you are looking for within the text.

- **Read Quickly and Strategically:**

Instead of reading every word, search for specific phrases or terms that match what you're looking for. This is because your goal is to quickly look through the text till you find the information you need.

- **Stay Focused:**

You cannot effectively scan any passage if you keep being distracted by unrelated details as you scan. So, ensure you keep your attention sharp and focused as you scan.

Just like other reading techniques, let's also apply scanning to a passage from the TEAS 7 examination. Here, you'll imagine that the passage is about the human body (anatomy) and you need to find information about the functions of the heart (respiratory system). To scan the passage effectively you'll need to:

→ Look for headings or sections that mention the heart/respiratory system.

→ Look for keywords like "lungs," "heart," "cardiovascular system," "breathing," "pumping blood," or "oxygen exchange" to guide your search.

→ Quickly read through the text and pay attention to sentences or phrases that talk about the heart's function or structure, such as "delivering oxygen to the bloodstream."

→ And once you've located the relevant information, you can now focus on understanding it in more detail or using it to answer questions about the heart (respiratory system).

Scanning is a reading technique that is so valuable when you need to quickly find specific details relevant for answering a question in the TEAS 7 exam.

➢ Annotation

Annotation is a powerful reading technique for anyone preparing for the TEAS 7 examination. Especially for the reading section. It is a way of actively interacting with the passage or material by writing notes, marking questions, observations, and important information. As a valuable tool that can significantly enhance your reading comprehension skills, annotation makes you think deeply about the text, make connections, and understand the topic better.

This is because, as you read, you are prompted to consider the author's main arguments, identify supporting evidence, and evaluate the overall structure and organization of the passage.

When you annotate, you're not just reading passively, instead you are writing down your thoughts and questions, creating connections and a personal record of the important insights gotten from the text. These annotations can serve as a useful reference when you are reviewing the material later on. It'll help you recall key points, clarify confusing passages, and deepen your understanding of the material.

To make effective annotations, you should:

- **Highlight Key Points:**

Underlining or highlighting important information in the passage is a great way to quickly identify the key points and central ideas. Annotations will also help you not to forget where key ideas or information are located as the highlighting colors and marks will easily pop them out. This, of course will help you easily pay attention to the most relevant details when reviewing the passage later.

- **Make Margin Notes:**

Margin notes are like your own personal study guide or reference note when you read. It is where you write short summaries, questions, or comments from the passage. You can always jot down points at the margin to help you understand the passage better and to make complex information simpler. It helps you ask questions that will clarify confusing parts and also organizes your thoughts as you read. Margin notes is also useful tool for studying and reviewing later on.

- **Identify Vocabulary:**

Annotation also allows you to identify and define unfamiliar vocabulary words directly within the text. With annotations, you can write the meaning or definitions of the words, or the synonyms alongside the word in the passage. It is important to identify new terms as you read, because they will give you a better understanding of the passage as well as help improve your reading comprehension skills.

- **Track Themes and Patterns:**

With annotation, you can track recurring themes, patterns, or motifs throughout the text. You'll also be able to note connections between different parts of the passage that will help you gain a deeper understanding of the author's message and intent. For example, you can connect a cause in the passage to it's implications, preventions, and solutions.

- **Create Visual Cues:**

You can use symbols, bullets, or arrows to annotate important parts of the passage while reading. This will draw your attention to specific passages or concepts within the text, thereby making any relevant information easier to find later.

- **Engaging with Complex Passages:**

Annotations help you break down difficult and challenging passages into paragraphs or sentences that you can easily understand. It helps you break the text into smaller, recognizable parts where you extract their meaning, messages, main ideas, supporting details, and transitions.

Now, let's apply what you've read so far. If you are reading a passage on cell biology. Here is a rundown on how you can annotate:

→ Skim the passage to get an overview of its content and structure. Look for headings or sections that mention cell structure or function.

→ As you read more closely, pay attention to keywords related to cell biology, such as "cell membrane," "nucleus," "organelles," and "mitochondria."

→ Use a pen or highlighter to mark any sentences or phrases that discuss important concepts or structures within the cell. For example, you might highlight a sentence that explains the role of the nucleus in controlling cellular activities.

→ In the margins of the text or on a separate piece of paper, jot down any questions you have about cell biology or any connections you notice between different parts of the passage.

→ After you've finished annotating the passage, take a moment to review your annotations. Reflect on the main ideas and key points you highlighted, as well as any insights you gained from your notes.

→ Finally, try to summarize the main idea or central theme of the passage related to cell biology based on your annotations. Also, write a short paragraph that captures the essence of what you've read, using your annotations as a guide.

In summary, annotating is one helpful reading technique that you should practice if you want to successfully understand your TEAS 7 examination subjects.

➤ Chunking

Chunking is when you take a large amount of information and break it down into smaller, easier-to-handle pieces. It is like organizing a messy closet into smaller, neatly arranged sections, in order to make it easier to find what you need.

This technique is particularly beneficial for you a TEAS 7 exam candidate, who needs to process and retain complex, lengthy, and challenging key concepts or information efficiently. Because it would help you understand and remember the complex information easily as well as make it easier for you to tackle challenging questions and tasks in the exam hall.

For example, with chunking, you can dissect or organize lengthy passages, mathematical problems, tough scientific topics, information and passages into smaller groups or categories that you handle. This make the study, problem solving or examination less overwhelming.

As a TEAS 7 student, you can effectively utilize chunking when reading by:

• Breaking Down Passages Into Parts:

When faced with lengthy passages in the Reading Comprehension section, you should break down the long passage into smaller and more manageable sections. You can do this perfectly by looking at where the story has different sections, paragraphs, and main ideas. Then you can focus on understanding one section at a time without feeling overwhelmed or confused by the entire passage.

- **Finding the Important Information:**

After breaking the passage into chunks, move on to find the main ideas, definitions, supporting details, and key vocabulary. This way you can grasp the essential information presented in the passage and also find answers to the exam questions.

- **Making Connections:**

As you read through each chunk of the passage, check for how each chunk of the story connects to the others. This way you will not miss any part and you'll understand the overall picture better.

- **Practicing with Questions:**

When answering questions related to the passage, use the chunking technique there too. Doing this makes it easier to find the right answer because you will be breaking break down the question stem and answer choices into smaller components that will allow you to analyze each part individually and eliminate incorrect options more efficiently.

Here is a rundown on how you can chunk easily. Imagine you're studying a passage about the human circulatory system for the TEAS 7 exam. Instead of trying to read the whole thing at once, you should:

→ Choose a section of the study material that discusses the components and functions of the circulatory system, such as the heart, blood vessels, and blood circulation.
→ Break the passage into smaller, manageable chunks of information. For example, you could separate the passage into sections focusing on the structure of the heart, the types of blood vessels, and the process of blood circulation.

→ Read one chunk at a time, focusing on understanding the main idea and key details.

→ After reading each chunk, summarize the information in your own words. For instance, summarize the function of the heart in pumping blood and the role of arteries, veins, and capillaries in transporting blood throughout the body.

→ As you progress through the passage, look for connections between the chunks. Identify how each chunk relates to the overall topic of the circulatory system and how the information builds upon previous sections.

→ Use your summaries to piece together the entire passage and understand the flow of information. Pay attention to how each chunk contributes to the broader concept of the circulatory system and its importance for human health.

→ After chunking the passage, test your comprehension by recalling the main points of each section without referring back to the text. This exercise will help reinforce your understanding and retention of the material.

It is also essential to note that chunking can help you manage your time more effectively during the exam. Because as you break down the passages and questions into smaller segments, you can allocate enough time which will enable you to carefully read and analyze each chunk without feeling rushed. Overall, applying chunking as a reading strategy can empower you to approach complex passages with more confidence and clarity.

➢ **Visualization**

Visualization is a reading technique where you create mental images or "movies" of the text as you read. This technique involves using your imagination to picture the scenes, characters, actions, and settings described in the passage or material.

When you engage your mind this way while reading, you enhance your comprehension of the text, you'll recall the information easily, and also enjoy reading the material, topic or passage.

As a TEAS 7 student, you can effectively apply visualization as a reading technique by:

- **Creating Mental Images:**

As you read a passage, actively visualize the scenes, characters, and actions described in the text. You'll need to imagine yourself within the setting of the passage, observing the events as they unfold. For example, if the passage describes a scene in a park, imagine yourself standing in that park, surrounded by trees, flowers, and people.

- **Engaging Your Senses:**

As you read, use your senses to enhance your mental images. Imagine the sights, sounds, smells, tastes, and textures associated with the passage. Let it be as if you were actually experiencing the events described in the passage. For example, if you're reading about a laboratory experiment, visualize the equipment, chemicals, and reactions taking place, and imagine the sounds of bubbling liquids and the smells of various substances. This imagery will make you never forget what the passage, material, or topic is all about.

- **Focusing on Details:**

You should also pay attention to the specific details mentioned in the text and use them to create vivid images in your mind. Notice the dates, items, colors, shapes, sizes, and movements described in the passage, and try to visualize them as vividly as possible.

- **Connect To Previous Knowledge or Personal Experiences:**

Try to relate the content of the passage to your own experiences, knowledge, and memories. Draw upon familiar concepts or situations that you may know about to enrich your mental images and deepen your understanding of the text. Also, use your imagination to fill in any gaps or ambiguities in the text.

If the passage doesn't provide a detailed description of a character or setting, use your imagination to create those details yourself.

- **Practice Visualization Exercises:**

To improve your visualization skills, you need to practice. You can start with short passages and gradually work your way up to longer and more complex texts. For example, read a short passage and then close your eyes to visualize the scene before attempting to recall the specific details from memory.

We've gotten to the rundown point. Here is a rundown on how you can visualize easily. Let's say you're reading a passage about the human circulatory system for the TEAS 7 exam. As you read, you come across a description of how blood flows through the heart and arteries. Instead of just reading the words on the page, you can:

→ Imagine yourself standing inside the heart, watching as blood is pumped in and out with each heartbeat.

→ Then visualize the arteries branching out from the heart like a network of roads, carrying oxygen-rich blood to every part of the body.

→ You can even imagine the blood cells themselves, flowing smoothly through the arteries like tiny cars on a highway.

Finally, this reading technique should be considered important because it can enhance your understanding and retention of the material read. Also, visual images are often easier to remember than words alone, so this technique can help you recall information more effectively when you need it for the TEAS 7 exam.

➢ **Summarization**

You can easily define summarization as taking a big piece of information, like a long passage or topic, and making it shorter while still keeping the main ideas.

It is like giving a brief overview or snapshot of the important parts of a passage, topic, or material without getting into all the small details. It involves extracting the most important elements of the text and presenting them in a clear and succinct manner. This is a valuable technique that helps you easily understand the essence of a passage quickly, without getting you bogged down by unnecessary details.

As a high-flying TEAS 7 student, you can apply summarization effectively by:

- **Identifying the Main Ideas:**

When reading a passage, focus on identifying the main ideas, supporting details, or central themes. Look for recurring concepts, key arguments, or important points that the author emphasizes throughout the text. Then, you can use your own words to concisely summarize the main points of the passage without including any unnecessary detail.

- **Using the "Five Ws and One H" Framework:**

One approach to summarizing is to use the "Who, What, When, Where, Why, and How" framework. These are questions used to gather information and understand the key aspects of a situation, event, or topic. As a TEAS 7 student, you should ask yourself these questions as you read. Then, use your answers to construct a brief summary of the passage. This framework ensures that you capture all the essential messages from the passage in your summary.

- **Paraphrasing the Information:**

Another strategy to summarize perfectly is to paraphrase the information in the passage, rephrasing it in a way that is clear and concise. Do not copy directly from the passage. You can do this by putting the main ideas and key details into your own words. The role of paraphrasing is to help you internalize the information and ensures that you understand it fully.

- **Organizing the Summary:**

Ensure you structure your summary in a logical manner that presents the main ideas in a clear and coherent sequence. Use headings, bullet points, or numbered lists to organize the information and make it easier to follow.

- **Checking for Accuracy:**

After writing your summary, you need to review it to ensure that you have accurately represented the main ideas and key details of the passage. Checking for accuracy will also lead you into making any necessary revisions that would improve the clarity of your summary.

Here is a brief rundown on how you can summarize perfectly. So, imagine you are reading a passage about the human brain and it is filled with scientific terms and complex explanations, making it seem like an insurmountable mountain of information. Instead of feeling overwhelmed, you should:

→ You read through each paragraph carefully, highlighting the main idea and key supporting details. For example, one paragraph discusses the different lobes of the brain and their functions: the frontal lobe for decision-making, the parietal lobe for sensory perception, and so on. Another paragraph explains how neurons transmit signals through electrical impulses.

→ After reading, you take a moment to reflect and synthesize the information. You jot down a concise summary in your own words: "The human brain is divided into different lobes, each responsible for specific functions like decision-making and sensory perception. Neurons are the cells that transmit signals in the brain, using electrical impulses."

Additionally, you can practice summarization by writing short summaries of passages you encounter during your study sessions. Being the last reading technique discussed in this book, it is important to to let you know that practicing summarization regularly will make you become more efficient at extracting key information from passages, which will in turn, help you succeed your TEAS 7 exam.

Key Idea Identification:
Strategies For Identifying Main Ideas And Key Points Within Reading Materials

Key idea identification means exactly what you think. But this time, you'll understand more indepthly what it means. It means finding the main points or central themes in a piece of writing. It is all about understanding what the author is trying to say. Which is the primary message or argument that is being conveyed.

This is important because it helps you grasp the core meaning, most important parts, and the purpose of the text. It's like finding the heart of the message so you can understand it better.

When it comes to reading comprehension, being able to grasp the main idea of a passage is essential. This is because the main idea encapsulates the central theme or argument that the author is conveying, providing readers with a clear understanding of the purpose and focus of the text.

You usually find this in the topic sentence or thesis statement at the start of a paragraph or passage. These sentences give you the main point in a clear and simple way.

Now, let's explore the strategies for identifying main ideas and key points within reading materials.

➢ Skimming and Scanning
Skimming as we've explained previously involves quickly glancing through the text to understand its overall gist, while scanning involves searching for specific information or keywords.

You can start by skimming the text to get an overview of the content. Look for headings, subheadings, and topic sentences to quickly grasp the main ideas of each section. This strategy is particularly useful for swiftly identifying main ideas and key points in time-sensitive situations like standardized tests like the TEAS 7 exam.

➤ Identify Topic Sentences

Topic sentences often serve as mini-summaries of paragraphs, encapsulating the main idea within a concise statement. By recognizing and understanding these sentences in the passage you can grasp the key ideas of each section or paragraph more easily.

➤ Look for Repetition

Additionally, pay attention to repetition or emphasis within the text. Authors often reinforce their main ideas by repeating key concepts or phrases throughout the text or by presenting them in a more prominent way. Look for recurring words, themes, keywords, or phrases that indicate important concepts as they are likely indicative of the central message the author wants to convey.

➤ Think Critically

Another strategy is to think critically and to actively engage with the text while reading. Ask yourself questions like, "What is the author trying to convey?" and "What are the main arguments or points being made?" Check out the author's purpose, perspective, and arguments.

Also consider the implications of the main ideas presented and how they relate to broader themes or contexts.
By actively questioning the text, you can better identify and comprehend the key ideas presented.

➤ Practice Summarizing

Summarizing the text in your own words can help solidify your understanding of the main ideas. Try to condense each paragraph or section into a concise summary that focuses on capturing the essence of the author's message.

➢ Context

Lastly, don't forget to consider the context of the reading material. Think about the bigger picture. Consider why the author wrote the text and who it is written for. Understanding this can give you clues about the main ideas. Understanding the purpose, audience, and context of the text provides you with valuable insights into the main ideas and key points being conveyed.

By using these strategies into your reading approach, you can better identify and understand the main ideas and key points in various reading materials. So, whether you're tackling passages on the TEAS 7 exam or delving into other academic or professional texts, these strategies will do the magic.

(Action Steps)
Exercises for Enhancing Reading Comprehension

Exercise One:
Reading Comprehension Practice Passage

Title: The Importance of Sleep

Getting an adequate amount of sleep is essential for overall health and well-being. Sleep plays a crucial role in various bodily functions, including cognitive function, emotional regulation, and physical recovery. Despite its importance, many individuals struggle to prioritize sleep in their daily routines, leading to detrimental effects on their health and productivity.

One of the primary functions of sleep is to support cognitive function and brain health. During sleep, the brain consolidates memories, processes information, and clears out toxins accumulated throughout the day.

Adequate sleep is particularly important for students preparing for exams, as it enhances learning and memory retention.

Furthermore, sleep is closely linked to emotional regulation and mental health. Sleep deprivation can lead to irritability, mood swings, and increased stress levels. Chronic sleep problems have been associated with a higher risk of developing mood disorders such as depression and anxiety. Prioritizing quality sleep can help individuals maintain emotional balance and resilience in the face of daily challenges.

In addition to cognitive and emotional benefits, sleep plays a critical role in physical health and recovery. During sleep, the body repairs tissues, synthesizes hormones, and regulates metabolic processes. Lack of sleep can compromise immune function, increase inflammation, and elevate the risk of chronic diseases such as obesity, diabetes, and cardiovascular disorders.

In conclusion, getting enough high-quality sleep is essential for overall health and well-being. By prioritizing sleep and adopting healthy sleep habits, individuals can optimize their cognitive function, emotional well-being, and physical health.

Comprehension Questions:

1. What is one primary function of sleep mentioned in the passage?
2. How does sleep deprivation affect emotional regulation?
3. Name one chronic disease associated with lack of sleep.
4. Why is adequate sleep particularly important for students preparing for exams?
5. How can individuals optimize their overall health and well-being according to the passage?
6. What's one important thing sleep does for your brain?
7. What's the main message of the passage about sleep?
8. How does not getting enough sleep affect your emotions?

Exercise Two:

Title: Mental Health

"In recent years, there has been growing awareness of the importance of mental health and well-being in overall health outcomes. Mental health is not merely the absence of mental illness, but rather a state of well-being in which individuals can cope with the normal stresses of life, work productively, and contribute to their communities.

However, mental health disorders, such as depression, anxiety, and bipolar disorder, affect millions of people worldwide and can have profound impacts on daily functioning and quality of life. Addressing mental health concerns requires a multifaceted approach, including access to mental health services, social support networks, and strategies for stress management and self-care.

By promoting mental health awareness and destigmatizing mental illness, communities can create environments that support positive mental health outcomes for all individuals."

Comprehension Questions:

1. What is the main focus of the passage?
2. How is mental health defined in the passage?
3. List three mental health disorders mentioned in the passage.
4. What factors contribute to mental health concerns, according to the passage?
5. How does the passage suggest addressing mental health concerns?
6. What role do communities play in promoting positive mental health outcomes, according to the passage?
7. Why is it important to destigmatize mental illness, based on the passage?
8. Describe the impact of mental health disorders on individuals, as mentioned in the passage.
9. What are some strategies mentioned in the passage for managing mental health?

10. How does the passage suggest creating environments supportive of positive mental health outcomes?

Chapter 4:

Math Skills Unlocked

In this chapter, we're going to focus on the important math concepts (arithmetic and algebra) as well as techniques for interpreting and analyzing data which you'll need to know for the TEAS exam. So whether you are a lover of maths or someone who finds numbers a bit challenging, this chapter will help you get ready for the math section of the TEAS test.

Mathematics plays a crucial role in many aspects of healthcare. From calculating medication dosages to understanding and interpreting medical research data, you an aspiring healthcare professional, must possess strong math skills to succeed in your academic studies and future healthcare career. That's where this chapter comes in. This chapter provides you with a comprehensive review of math fundamentals tailored to the specific requirements of the TEAS exam.

This entire chapter will cover everything from basic arithmetic operations like addition, subtraction, multiplication, and division to more complex algebraic equations. We will also explore the different methods for understanding, interpreting and analyzing data presented in various formats, like tables, graphs, and charts. So whether you are brushing up on your math skills or starting from scratch, we are here to guide you every step of the way. Now, let's get started and unlock your math potential for success on the TEAS exam!

Fundamentals of Arithmetic and Algebra:

Explanations on Essential Maths Concepts and Problem-Solving Methods

We'll begin this section by reviewing the four fundamental arithmetic concepts/operations, that is: addition, subtraction, multiplication, and division. Understanding these concepts is important because they form the basis for any other complex math problem that you may come across in the TEAS 7 examination. We'll break down each operation step by step for you and we'll practice with you by solving different maths problems on this. This way you can get a solid grasp of these foundational concepts.

➤ Addition

Addition is one of the fundamental arithmetic operations and it is used to find the total sum of two or more numbers. In simpler terms, it involves putting numbers together to find out how much there is in total.

In mathematical notation, the addition symbol is represented by the plus sign (+). For example, if you have 2 apples and you buy 3 more, you can find out how many apples you have in total by adding the numbers together: 2 + 3 = 5 apples.

One thing you should know about addition is that it follows several important properties and they include the commutative property (which says that changing the order of numbers does not change the sum), the associative property (says changing the grouping of numbers doesn't change the sum), and the identity property (says that adding zero to any number doesn't change the value of that number).

Now, in the context of the TEAS 7 exam, the addition arithmetic operation plays a crucial role in various aspects of the TEAS 7 exam, especially in scenarios related to real-life applications such as medication administration and budgeting. In medication administration, nurses and healthcare professionals often need to calculate dosages accurately to ensure the patient safety.

Which is where the addition knowledge comes into play as they must calculate the total dosage needed based on factors like patient weight, medication concentration, and prescribed dosage per kilogram. For example, if a medication is prescribed at 2 milligrams per kilogram of body weight, and the patient weighs 70 kilograms, you would need to add the total dosage required based on this calculation.

Similarly, in budget scenarios, addition is important for determining total costs and expenses. For instance, if you're creating a household budget or managing expenses for a project, you'll need to add up various expenses such as rent or mortgage payments, utility bills, groceries, transportation costs, and entertainment expenses to calculate the total amount you are spending within a given time frame.

This two scenarios depict that accuracy and efficiency is key because on the TEAS 7 exam day, you will encounter questions that require you to perform additions quickly and accurately, as well as to solve addition problems within a limited time frame.

Therefore, being good at addition means you can solve these kinds of problems easily and without mistakes. This is important to successfully pass the TEAS 7 exam. So, practicing and familiarizing yourself with different types addition problems will help you get better at it, build confidence, and tackle the questions with ease on the exam day.

Moving on to examples of how you can solve addition problems, here are the various types of addition problems that a TEAS 7 student may encounter, ranging from basic arithmetic to more complex scenarios involving decimals, fractions, and real-world situations. Try doing this in five minutes.

- **Simple Whole Number Addition:**
  - Add 25 and 17.
  - Solution: 25 + 17 = 42

Here, we simply add 25 and 17 together to get 42 as the sum.

- **Addition with Decimals:**
  - Add 3.6 and 2.8.
  - Solution: 3.6 + 2.8 = 6.4

    Adding 3.6 and 2.8 results in a sum of 6.4.

- **Addition with Fractions:**
  - Add 3/4 and 1/3.
  - Solution: (3/4) + (1/3) = (9/12) + (4/12) = 13/12

To add fractions, we first find a common denominator, then add the numerators. In this case, 3/4 plus 1/3 equals 13/12.

- **Addition of Negative Numbers:**
  - Add -5 and -8.
  - Solution: -5 + (-8) = -13

    When adding negative numbers, we combine their absolute values first and keep the double negative sign.

- **Real-World Addition Problem:**
  - If you have $15 and you earn $20, how much money do you have in   total?
  - Solution: $15 + $20 = $35

    Adding $15 and $20 together gives a total of $35.

- **Estimation Addition Problem:**

  Estimate this sum before calculating:
  - 158 + 92
  - Solution: To estimate the sum of 158 and 92, we can round each number to the nearest tens:
  - 158 rounds to 160.
  - 92 rounds to 90.
  - Now, adding 160 and 90 gives us an estimated sum of 250.
  - So, the estimated sum of 158 + 92 is 250.

Now that you've seen these examples, try doing these addition exercises in 15 minutes. Remember the TEAS 7 examination is not about solving alone but about timing. So set the Timer and Solve!

<u>*Action Steps:*</u>

Addition Speed Drill

Set a timer for 15 minutes and see how many addition problems you can solve correctly within the time limit.

- **Basic Addition Practice:**

Calculate the sum of the following pairs of numbers:

a) 25 + 13
b) 47 + 29
c) 82 + 16
d) 63 + 54

- **Addition with Decimals:**

- Add 4.7 and 6.25.
- Add 8.36 and 3.82.

- **Addition with Fractions:**

- Add 5/6 and 2/5.
- Add 7/8 and 3/10.

- **Addition of Negative Numbers:**

- Add -12 and -9.
- Add -7 and -15.

- **Word Problem Practice:**

Solve the following word problems involving addition:

a) A research lab conducted experiments over three consecutive days. On the first day, they conducted 345 trials, on the second day, 429 trials, and on the third day, 511 trials. How many trials did the lab conduct in total over the three days?

b) A pharmaceutical company received shipments of medication from two suppliers. The first supplier delivered 768 boxes of pills, while the second supplier delivered 586 boxes. If each box contains 100 pills, how many pills did the company receive in total from both suppliers?

c) A hospital received emergency patients throughout the day. In the morning, they received 152 patients, in the afternoon, they received 189 patients, and in the evening, they received 231 patients. How many emergency patients did the hospital receive in total for the day?

- **Multi-digit Addition Practice**:

Perform the following multi-digit additions:

a) 326 + 158

b) 497 + 234

c) 815 + 429

d) 673 + 567

- **Estimation Practice:**

Estimate the sum of the following pairs of numbers before calculating:

a) 146 + 98

b) 279 + 354

c) 528 + 177

d) 413 + 689

➤ **Subtraction**

Subtraction is the process of taking away one number from another to find the difference between them. When you're subtracting, the number from which another number is subtracted is called the minuend, while the number being subtracted is called the subtrahend. The result of the subtraction is called the difference.

For example, if you have 8 apples and you eat 3 of them, you are performing a subtraction operation: 8 (minuend) - 3 (subtrahend) = 5 (difference). This means that after eating 3 apples, you have 5 apples remaining.

In addition to basic subtraction, there are also different strategies and techniques that can be used to solve subtraction problems more efficiently. Some of these include regrouping or borrowing when subtracting larger numbers. These, make use of mental math strategies like counting backwards or using number bonds, as well as applying estimation to check the reasonableness of the result.

Furthermore, subtraction is often used in conjunction with other arithmetic operations, such as addition, multiplication, and division, to solve more complex problems such as the multi-step word problem. Here, you may need to use subtraction to find the difference between two quantities before using that information in further calculations.

Moving on to examples of how you can solve subtraction problems, here are the various types of subtraction problems that a TEAS 7 student may encounter and they range from basic arithmetic to more complex scenarios involving decimals, fractions, and real-world problems.

- **Basic Whole Number Subtraction:**
  - Subtract 38 from 72.
  - Solution: 72 - 38 = 34
    Subtracting 38 from 72 leaves 34 as the difference.

- **Subtraction with Decimals:**
  - Subtract 5.6 from 9.2.
  - Solution: 9.2 - 5.6 = 3.6
    Subtracting 5.6 from 9.2 results in a difference of 3.6.

- **Subtraction with Fractions:**
  - Subtract 3/5 from 1.
  - Solution: 1 - 3/5 = 5/5 - 3/5 = 2/5
    To subtract fractions, we find a common denominator and then subtract the numerators. Here, 1 minus 3/5 equals 2/5.

- **Subtraction of Negative Numbers:**
- Subtract -10 from -5.
- Solution: -5 - (-10) = -5 + 10 = 5

When subtracting a negative number, it's like adding its absolute value. So, -5 minus (-10) equals -5 plus 10, which is 5.

- **Multi-Step Word Problem Involving Subtraction**

A bakery sells 150 cupcakes each day. If 30 cupcakes were sold in the morning and 45 were sold in the afternoon, how many cupcakes were sold in the evening?

- Solution: To find out how many cupcakes were sold in the evening, you'll subtract the combined morning and afternoon sales from the total daily sales.

First, you'll calculate the total number of cupcakes sold in the morning and afternoon:
- Morning sales: 30 cupcakes
- Afternoon sales: 45 cupcakes
- Total morning and afternoon sales: 30 + 45 = 75 cupcakes

Then you'll subtract the total morning and afternoon sales from the total daily sales to find the evening sales:
- Total daily sales: 150 cupcakes
- Evening sales: 150 - 75 = 75 cupcakes

Now that you've seen these examples, try doing these in 15 minutes. Remember the TEAS 7 examination is not about solving alone but about timing. So set the Timer and Solve!

Action Steps:
Subtraction Speed Drill

Set a timer for 15 minute and see how many subtraction problems you can solve correctly within the time limit.

- **Basic Subtraction:**
  - 8 - 3 =
  - 15 - 7 =
  - 42 - 19 =

- **Subtraction with Regrouping/Borrowing:**
  - **54 - 28 =**
  - 93 - 47 =
  - 326 - 158 =

- **Subtraction with Decimals:**
- Subtract 19.37 from 54.68.
- Subtract 73.21 from 98.54.

- **Subtraction with Fractions:**
- Subtract 7/8 from
- Subtract 5/6 from 1 2/3.

- **Subtraction of Negative Numbers:**
- Subtract -28 from -15.
- Subtract -14 from -6.

- **Multi-step Word Problems Involving Subtraction:**
Solve the following word problems involving addition
a) A hospital has 256 patients admitted to the emergency room. Throughout the day, 148 patients were discharged. How many patients are still in the emergency room?
b) A bookstore had 539 books in stock at the beginning of the month. During the month, 287 books were sold, and 62 books were returned by customers. How many books are left in the bookstore's inventory at the end of the month?

c) A construction company purchased 375 bags of cement for a project. After completing half of the project, they realized they only needed 214 bags of cement. How many bags of cement are left unused?

d) During a sale, a department store had 892 shirts in stock. Over the course of the sale, 367 shirts were sold, and 128 new shirts were added to the inventory. How many shirts are now in stock at the department store?

➤ Multiplication

Multiplication is the process of combining groups of numbers to find a total or product. It's like adding a number to itself several times. For example, 3 multiplied by 4 means adding 3 four times: 3 + 3 + 3 + 3, which equals 12.

In multiplication, one number is called the multiplicand, another number is called the multiplier, and the result is called the product. Also, it is often represented using the multiplication symbol "×" or by writing the numbers next to each other, like 3 × 4 = 12.

You can use multiplication in various real-life situations, like calculating prices when buying multiple items, finding the total number of items in several equal groups, or determining the area of a rectangle.

Now, to examples of how you can solve multiplication problems, here are the various types of multiplication problems that a TEAS 7 student may encounter and they range from basic arithmetic to more complex scenarios involving decimals, fractions, and real-world problems.

- **Simple Whole Number Multiplication:**
  - Multiply 7 by 8.
  - Solution: 7 × 8 = 56
    Multiplying 7 by 8 equals 56.

- **Multiplication with Decimals:**
  - Multiply 3.2 by 4.5.

- Solution: 3.2 × 4.5 = 14.4
  Multiplying 3.2 by 4.5 results in 14.4.

- **Multiplication with Fractions:**
- Multiply 2/3 by 5/6.
- Solution: (2/3) × (5/6) = 10/18 = 5/9

To multiply fractions, we multiply the numerators and denominators separately. Here, (2/3) multiplied by (5/6) equals 10/18, which simplifies to 5/9.

- **Multiplication of Mixed Numbers:**
- Multiply 2 1/2 by 3 1/4.
- Solution: (2 1/2) × (3 1/4) = 2.5 × 3.25 = 8.125

To multiply mixed numbers, we first convert them to improper fractions, then multiply them. Here, (2 1/2) multiplied by (3 1/4) equals 8.125.

- **Real-World Multiplication Problem:**
- If each book costs $15 and you buy 5 books, how much do you spend?
- Solution: 15 × 5 = $75

Multiplying the cost per book ($15) by the number of books (5) results in a total of $75.

Now that you've seen these examples, try doing these in 15 minutes. Remember the TEAS 7 examination is not about solving alone but about timing. So set the Timer and Solve!

Action Steps:
Multiplication Speed Drill

Set a timer for 15 minute and see how many subtraction problems you can solve correctly within the time limit.

- **Simple Whole Number Multiplication:**

a) $7 \times 9 =$

b) $5 \times 8 =$

c) $126 \times 84 =$

d) $597 \times 23 =$

- **Multiplication with Decimals:**

a) $2.3 \times 4.5 =$

b) $6.78 \times 3.2 =$

- **Multiplication with Fractions:**

a) Multiply 3/4 by 5/8

b) Multiply 2/5 by 4/7

- **Multiplication of Mixed Numbers:**

a) Multiply 1 2/3 by 2 3/4

b) Multiply 3 4/5 by 1 1/2

- **Real-World Multiplication Problem:**

a) A software company releases updates every 3 months, each update consisting of 6 new features. If the company has been releasing updates for 5 years, how many features have they introduced in total?

b) If a car travels at a speed of 65 miles per hour for 4 hours, how far does it travel?

c) A recipe calls for 3 cups of flour, and you need to make 5 batches of the recipe. How many cups of flour do you need in total?

d) A carpenter needs to cut 36 boards into equal lengths. If each board is 8 feet long and the carpenter can cut 3 boards at a time, how many cuts will be needed in total?

➢ **Division**

Division is the process of splitting a number into equal parts or groups. It's the opposite of multiplication. In division, you have a dividend, which is the total number you want to divide, a divisor, which is the number you are dividing by, and a quotient, which is the result of the division.

For example, if you have 12 cookies and you want to divide them equally among 3 friends, you would perform the division operation 12 ÷ 3. Here, 12 is the dividend, 3 is the divisor, and the quotient would be 4, meaning each friend would get 4 cookies.

In the TEAS 7 exam, you may find division problems in various scenarios, such as distributing items equally, calculating rates or ratios, or finding the remainder after dividing.

Now, to examples of how you can solve multiplication problems, here are the various types of division problems that a TEAS 7 student may encounter and they range from basic arithmetic to more complex scenarios involving decimals, fractions, and real-world problems.

- **Simple Whole Number Division:**
  - Divide 20 by 5.
  - Solution: $20 ÷ 5 = 4$

  In this case, the dividend is 20, and the divisor is 5. The quotient, or the result of the division, is 4.

- **Division with Remainder:**
  - Divide 17 by 4.
  - Solution: $17 ÷ 4 = 4$ with a remainder of 1

  In this example, 17 is divided by 4. The quotient is 4, and the remainder is 1, meaning that after distributing 4 equally, there is 1 left over.

- **Division with Decimals:**
  - Divide 8.4 by 2.
  - Solution: $8.4 ÷ 2 = 4.2$

  Here, we divide 8.4 by 2, resulting in a quotient of 4.2.

- **Division with Fractions:**

 - Divide 3/4 by 1/2.
 - Solution: $(3/4) \div (1/2) = (3/4) \times (2/1) = 3/2 = 1\,1/2$

To divide fractions, we multiply the first fraction by the reciprocal of the second fraction. In this case, (3/4) divided by (1/2) equals 3/2 or 1 1/2.

- **Real-World Division Problem:**

 - If a recipe calls for 2 cups of flour to make 12 cookies, how many cups of flour are needed to make 36 cookies?
 - Solution: 36 cookies ÷ 12 cookies = 3

Since the ratio of cookies to flour remains the same, you need 3 times the original amount of flour to make 36 cookies. So, you would need 3 cups of flour.

Now that you've seen these examples, try doing these in 15 minutes. Remember the TEAS 7 examination is not about solving alone but about timing. So set the Timer and Solve!

Action Steps:
Division Speed Drill

Set a timer for 15 minute and see how many subtraction problems you can solve correctly within the time limit.

- **Simple Whole Number Division:**

a) 789 ÷ 13 =
b) 1467 ÷ 21 =
c) 2156 ÷ 32 =

- **Division with Remainders:**

a) 103 ÷ 12 =
b) 285 ÷ 17 =

c) 462 ÷ 23 =

- **Division of Decimals:**

a) 8.64 ÷ 0.6 =
b) 15.12 ÷ 1.2 =
c) 23.76 ÷ 2.8 =

- **Division with Fractions:**

a) Divide 4/5 by 2/3.
b) Divide 5/6 by 3/4.

- **Word Problems Involving Division:**

a) If there are 364 students in a school and they need to be divided into 7 groups with an equal number of students in each group, how many students will be in each group?

b) A factory produces 3780 toys in a week. If the toys need to be packaged in boxes of 45 toys each, how many boxes are needed?

c) A factory produces 2400 widgets in a day. If the widgets are packaged into boxes containing 24 widgets each, how many boxes need to be filled in a day?

d) A group of students collected a total of 1080 books for a charity book drive. If the books are to be distributed equally among 15 schools, how many books will each school receive?

Algebra

Next, we will be exploring the algebraic concept and of course, it involves working with variables and solving equations. In this sub-section, you'll learn how to solve algebraic expressions, linear equations, and apply algebraic principles to real-world problems.

Learning how to solve algebra equations accurately and quickly is an important skill which you'll need for your TEAS 7 examination because you'll be asked many questions that will require you to set up and solve equations inorder to find the correct answer.

Algebra is a branch of mathematics that deals with symbols, variables, and the rules for manipulating them to solve equations and express relationships between quantities. It involves solving equations, working with variables, and manipulating algebraic expressions to analyze mathematical problems.

Algebra is all about using letters (like x or y) to stand for numbers and figuring out how they relate to each other. You also use rules to move these letters around, solve problems, and find out what the numbers are.

Algebraic concepts are widely used in various fields, including science, engineering, economics, and computer science, to model and solve real-world problems. In the context of the TEAS 7 exam, algebraic concepts are essential tools for solving equations, inequalities, and word problems.

Now just like life is governed by rules, Algebra uses rules to produce the right results and answers. There are several laws and properties that govern the manipulation and simplification of algebraic expressions and they include:

- **Commutative Property:**

This property states that changing the order of the terms in an addition or multiplication expression does not change the result. That is, you can change the order of numbers when you add or multiply them, and the result will stay the same.

For addition, it is expressed as (a + b = b + a), and for multiplication, it is (a times b = b times a). For example, 2 + 3 is the same as 3 + 2, and 2 × 3 is the same as 3 × 2.

- **Associative Property:**

This property states that the grouping of terms in an addition or multiplication expression does not change the result.

That simply means that, you can group numbers differently when you add or multiply them, and the result remains unchanged.

For addition, it is expressed as $((a + b) + c = a + (b + c))$, and for multiplication, it is $((a \times b) \times c = a \times (b \times c))$. For example, $(2 + 3) + 4$ is the same as $2 + (3 + 4)$, and $(2 \times 3) \times 4$ is the same as $2 \times (3 \times 4)$.

- **Distributive Property:**

This property allows us to distribute a factor across the terms inside parentheses. It let's you multiply a number by a group of numbers added together.

It also states that $(a \times (b + c) = a \times b + a \times c)$. For instance, if you have 2 multiplied by the sum of 3 and 4, it's the same as 2 multiplied by 3 plus 2 multiplied by 4.

- **Identity Property:**

The identity property for addition states that adding zero to any number leaves the number unchanged and expressed as $(a + 0 = a)$. This means, when you add zero to a number, it doesn't change the number.

The identity property for multiplication also states that multiplying any number by one leaves the number unchanged and expressed as $(a \times 1 = a)$. For example, $5 + 0$ is still 5, and 6×1 is still 6.

- **Inverse Property:**

The inverse property for addition states that adding the opposite of a number to the number results in zero and it is expressed as $(a + (-a) = 0)$.

Also, the inverse property for multiplication states that multiplying a number by its reciprocal results in one. For instance, adding a number to its opposite results in zero, and multiplying a number by its reciprocal gives one.

Try going over these five laws as many times as possible because when you understand and apply them, they will help you simplify algebraic expressions efficiently and accurately.

After talking about the rules, the next thing to talk about are some key algebraic concepts that every TEAS 7 students should be familiar with. *These algebraic concepts include:*

➤ **Variables:**

Variables are symbols (usually letters) that represent unknown quantities or values in mathematical expressions or equations. The most commonly used variables include x, y, a, b, and z.

In equations like $3x - 5 = 10$, the x is the mystery number we're trying to find. We can do math with variables, like adding, subtracting, multiplying, or dividing them.

Working with Variables:

There are different steps to efficiently solve variables which we have simplified for you.

The steps include:

- ***Step 1: Identify the Variables:***

Look for letters or symbols in the expression or equation that represent unknown quantities.

- ***Step 2: Combine Like Terms:***

If the expression contains similar terms with the same variables, combine them together. Like terms have the same variable(s) raised to the same power(s).

- ***Step 3: Apply the Order of Operations and Solve the Variable:***

If the expression or equation involves solving for a specific variable, isolate that variable by performing inverse operations. Perform the operations within the parentheses first, then apply the order of operations (PEMDAS: Parentheses, Exponents, Multiplication and Division from left to right, Addition and Subtraction from left to right) to simplify the expression.

- ● *Step 4: Substitute Values and Check Your Solution:*

After finding the value of the variable, substitute it back into the original expression or equation to verify its result's and its correctness.

Example 1:

Let's work with the expression $(3x - 2y + 4x + y)$.

- ➜ Identify the variables: x and y.
- ➜ Combine like terms: $3x$ and $4x$ are like terms, as well as $-2y$ and y. So, $3x + 4x = 7x$ and $-2y + y = -y$.
- ➜ Combine all the like terms together: $7x - y$.
- ➜ No specific values are given for x and y, so we leave the expression as $7x - y$.

Example 2:

Consider the expression $(3x + 2y - 5x + 4y)$ where $x = 2$ and $y = 3$.

- ➜ Identify the variables x and y.
- ➜ Simplify the expression by combining like terms: $$3x - 5x + 2y + 4y = (3 - 5)x + (2 + 4)y = -2x + 6y$$
- ➜ We're not solving for a specific variable here, but if we were, we'd isolate it using inverse operations.
- ➜ Check the solution by substituting $x = 2$ and $y = 3$ back into the simplified expression: $$-2(2) + 6(3) = -4 + 18 = 14$$

The result confirms our expression's correctness.

Example 3:

Suppose we have the expression $(2x + 3y - x + 5y)$. We want to simplify this expression by combining like terms.

→ In this expression, we have the variables x and y.
→ In our expression, the terms with the same variables can be combined together. So we have:
- $2x$ and $-x$ are like terms because they both have x.
- $3y$ and $5y$ are also like terms because they both have y.
→ Let's combine these like terms:
- $2x - x = x$ (Since $2x - x = 2x + (-x)$)
- $3y + 5y = 8y$ (Since $3y + 5y = 3y + 5y$)
→ Now that we've combined the like terms, let's put everything together:
- $(x + 8y)$

That's it! We've simplified the expression $(2x + 3y - x + 5y)$ to $(x + 8y)$. This means that if we were to substitute any specific values for x and y, we would use the simplified expression $(x + 8y)$.

(Action Steps)
Working With Variables

If you've gone through these three examples, it is wise to practice these exercises on variables using the steps we explained earlier.

Exercise 1:
Simplify the following algebraic expressions by combining like terms:

a) $(5x - 3y + 2x + 4y)$
b) $(2a + 3b - 4a + 5b)$

Exercise 2:
Given the expression $(4x - 2y = 10)$, solve for x when $y = 3$.

Exercise 3:
Simplify the following algebraic expressions by combining like terms:

a) $(2x + 3y - 4x + 5y)$
b) $(4a - 2b + 3a + 6b)$
c) If $(x = 3)$ and $(y = 2)$, find the value of $(4x - 2y + 5x)$.
d) If $(a = 5)$ and $(b = 2)$, find the value of $(2a - 3b + 2a + b)$.

➢ Equations
In algebra, equations are like balances - they show that two things are equal. They are mathematical statements expressing the equality of two expressions.

Solving equations simply means figuring out what number makes the equation true and the process involves using algebraic techniques such as isolating the variable, applying inverse operations, and simplifying expressions. For example, if we have $(2x + 3 = 11)$, we need to find the value of (x) that makes the equation correct.

Solving Equations:
There are different steps to efficiently solve equations and we have simplified them for you.

The steps include:

- ### Step 1: Look for the Variable
Find the letter or symbol (usually (x), (y), or (z)) that represents the unknown number.
- ### Step 2: Move the Numbers
If there are any numbers or terms next to the variable, move them to the other side of the equation using the opposite/inverse operation which says that addition becomes subtraction, and vice versa.
- ### Step 3: Isolate the Variable:

Once the numbers are on the other side, perform the opposite operation to isolate the variable. For example, if the variable is multiplied by a number, divide both sides by that number.

- ***Step 4: Check Your Answer:***

After finding the value of the variable, plug it back into the original equation to make sure it's correct.

Example 1:

Let's solve the equation $3y - 7 = 2y + 5$.

→ Look for the variable, which is y.
→ Move the numbers to the same side. Subtract $2y$ from both sides and add 7 to both sides: $3y - 2y = 5 + 7$
→ Combine like terms: $y = 12$
→ Check the answer. Plug $y = 12$ back into the original equation:
$3(12) - 7 = 2(12) + 5$
$36 - 7 = 24 + 5$
$29 = 29$

Since both sides are equal, our answer, $y = 12$, is correct!

Example 2:

Let's solve the equation $4x - 10 = 2x + 6$.

→ Look for the variable, which is x.
→ Move the numbers to the other side. Subtract $2x$ from both sides: $4x - 2x = 6 + 10$.
→ Simplify both sides: $2x = 16$.
→ Isolate the variable. Divide both sides by 2: $x = \frac{16}{2}$.
Solve for x: $x = 8$.

→ Check the answer. Plug $(x = 8)$ back into the original equation: $(4(8) - 10 = 2(8) + 6)$.

$$32 - 10 = 16 + 6$$
$$22 = 22$$

Since both sides are equal, our answer, $(x = 8)$, is correct!

(Action Steps)
Solving Equations

If you've gone through these examples, it is wise to practice these exercises on equations using the steps we explained earlier.

Solve the following equations:

1. Solve for (x): $(3x - 5 = 2x + 9)$.
2. Solve for (y): $(4y + 7 = 2(3y - 1))$.
3. Solve for (z): $(2(z + 3) - 5 = 3(z - 1))$.
4. Solve for (a): $(5(a - 4) + 2 = 3(a + 1) - 7)$.
5. Solve for (b): $(2(b - 5) + 3 = 4(b + 2) - 1)$.
6. Solve for (x): $(2x + 3 = 11)$.

➤ **Basic Algebraic Expressions**

Algebraic expressions are like math phrases. They combine numbers, variables (the mystery numbers), and math operations like adding or multiplying.

Simply put: An algebraic expression is a combination of numbers, variables, and arithmetic operations (such as addition, subtraction, multiplication, and division).

You need to understand how to work with these expressions, as they fundamental in solving algebraic equations and performing various mathematical operations.

For example, $(2x^2 + 3x - 5)$ is an expression with a variable (x) and some numbers.

Furthermore, the "^" symbol in mathematics indicates exponentiation, which means raising a number or variable to a certain power. For example, (x^2) means "x squared," indicating that (x) is multiplied by itself, resulting in (x) raised to the power of 2. Similarly, (x^3) would mean "x cubed," indicating that (x) is multiplied by itself twice, resulting in (x) raised to the power of 3.

Understanding Basic Algebraic Expressions:
There are different steps to understand and efficiently solve algebraic expressions and we have simplified them for you.

The steps include:

- ***Identify the Terms:***

In an algebraic expression, terms are separated by addition or subtraction signs. Each term can contain constants, variables, or both. Identify and isolate each term within the expression.

- ***Combine Like Terms:***

Like terms are terms that have the same variables raised to the same power. Combine these like terms together by performing the indicated arithmetic operations.

- ***Use the Order of Operations:***

Follow the order of operations (PEMDAS: Parentheses, Exponents, Multiplication and Division from left to right, Addition and Subtraction from left to right) to simplify the expression further. First, do any math inside parentheses. Then, work with exponents. After that, do multiplication and division. Finally, add or subtract.

- ***Evaluate the Expression:***

If you know what the values stand for, substitute those values into the expression and evaluate to find the result.

Example 1:

Let's work with the expression $(3x^2 + 2x - 5x + 7)$.

- → The terms are $3x^2$, $2x$, $-5x$, and 7.
- → $2x$ and $-5x$ are like terms, so we can combine them to get $-3x$. So, the expression becomes $3x^2 - 3x + 7$.
- → There are no parentheses or exponents to simplify further.
- → If specific values are given for x, we can substitute them into the expression and evaluate.

Example 2:

Let's work with the expression $(2a^3 + 4a^2b - 3ab^2 + 5b^3)$.

- → The terms are $2a^3$, $4a^2b$, $-3ab^2$, and $5b^3$.
- → There are no like terms in this expression since each term has different variables raised to different powers.
- → There are no parentheses or exponents to simplify further.
- → If specific values are given for a and b, we can substitute them into the expression and evaluate.

Example 3:

Let's work with the expression $(2(3x + 5) - 4(2x - 3))$.

- → The terms in this expression are $2(3x + 5)$, $-4(2x - 3)$.
- → There are no like terms that can be combined in this expression.

➜ We need to apply the distributive property first by multiplying each term outside the parentheses by each term inside the parentheses.

$$[2(3x + 5) = 6x + 10]$$
$$[-4(2x - 3) = -8x + 12]$$

➜ Now, we can combine the terms:

$$[6x + 10 - 8x + 12]$$
$$[= (6x - 8x) + (10 + 12)]$$
$$[= -2x + 22]$$

In this example, step 3 (using the order of operations) and step 4 (evaluating the expression) are effective because we have parentheses to simplify using the distributive property and combining like terms, respectively.

(Action Steps)
Basic Algebraic Expressions

If you've gone through these examples, it is wise to practice these exercises on expressions using the steps we explained earlier.

Exercise 1:

Simplify the following algebraic expressions:
a) $(3x + 2y - x + 4y)$
b) $(2a - 3b + 5a + 2b)$

Exercise 2:

Evaluate the following algebraic expressions for $(x = 4)$ *and* $(y = 2)$:
a) $(2x^2 - 3xy + y^2)$
b) $(3x + 4y - 2xy)$

Exercise 3:
Simplify the algebraic expression
a) $(3(2x - 4) + 5(3x + 2))$
b) $(2(x + 3) - 4(2x - 5))$

> **Inequalities**

In algebra, inequalities are like equations, but instead of saying two things are equal, they show a relationship between numbers using symbols like $(<)$, $(>)$, $(\leq)$, or $(\geq)$. Simply put: They are used to represent relationships where one quantity is greater than, less than, or not equal to another.

The symbol "≥" is read as "greater than or equal to $(\geq)$" and it represents a relationship between two quantities where the first quantity is either greater than or equal to the second quantity. In mathematical terms, it signifies that the value on the left side of the symbol is greater than or equal to the value on the right side.

Moving on, the term "leq" stands for "less than or equal to" and it is used in mathematical notation to represent an inequality where one value is less than or equal to another. The symbol for "leq" looks like this: "≤".

For instance, $(x < 5)$ means (x) is less than 5. it means that (x) can be any value less than or equal to 5. In other words, (x) can be 5 or any number less than 5. Solving these inequalities means finding the values of (x) that make the inequality true and it is just like solving equations.

As a TEAS 7 student, your questions involving inequalities may represent real-world scenarios or to compare quantities. This is because students use inequalities to determine ranges of values that satisfy certain conditions or constraints. For example, in a question about dosage limits for medication, students might use inequalities to ensure that the dosage falls within a safe range.

Solving Inequalities:

There are various steps to efficiently solve inequalities and we have simplified them for you.

The steps include:

- **Determine the Inequality Sign:**

Determine whether the inequality represents "greater than" (>), "less than" (<), "greater than or equal to" ($\geq$), or "less than or equal to" ($\leq$) relationships.

You need to pay attention to the direction of the inequality sign when performing operations and remember that multiplying or dividing both sides by a negative number will reverse the inequality sign.

- **Isolate the Variable:**

Similar to equations, start by getting the variable alone on one side of the inequality sign. Then, use inverse operations (opposite of addition, subtraction, multiplication, or division) to move terms to the other side.

- **Simplify and Solve the Variable:**

Once the variable is isolated, simplify the expression to find the possible values that satisfy the inequality. If there are variables on both sides of the inequality, move them to one side before simplifying.

- **Graph the Solution:**

Represent or draw the solution using interval notation on a number line or coordinate plane to visualize all the range of values that satisfy the inequality.

Example 1:

Let's solve the inequality $(2x + 3 > 7)$.

➜ The inequality sign is "greater than" (>).

→ Isolate the variable by subtracting 3 from both sides to isolate $2x$.
$$2x + 3 - 3 > 7 - 3$$
$$2x > 4$$

→ Solve the variable by dividing both sides by 2 to find the value of x.
$$\frac{2x}{2} > \frac{4}{2}$$
$$x > 2$$

→ Represent the solution $x > 2$ on a number line with an open circle at 2 and shade the region to the right to indicate all values greater than 2.

This example shows how to solve a basic inequality and represent its solution graphically.

Example 2:

Let's solve the inequality $2x + 3 > 7$.

→ Subtract 3 from both sides to isolate $2x$: $2x > 4$.
→ Since we divided both sides by a positive number (2), the direction of the inequality sign remains unchanged.
→ Divide both sides by 2 to solve for x: $x > 2$.
→ On a number line, we shade the region to the right of 2, indicating that any number greater than 2 is a solution.

Example 3:

Solve the real world application inequality problem:

a) A patient's heart rate must remain within 60 to 100 beats per minute. Write an inequality to represent this heart rate range, and determine if a heart rate of 85 beats per minute is within the acceptable range.

Inequality: $(60 < \{heart\ rate\} < 100)$

Explanation of Steps:

- **Identify the Range:**

The acceptable heart rate range is given as 60 to 100 beats per minute.

- **Write the Inequality:**

Use the symbols $\leq$ (less than or equal to) and $\geq$ (greater than or equal to) to represent the range. The inequality $60 \leq \text{heart rate} \leq 100$ means the heart rate must be greater than or equal to 60 beats per minute and less than or equal to 100 beats per minute.

- **Check the Heart Rate:**

Substitute the given heart rate (85 beats per minute) into the inequality to see if it falls within the acceptable range.

- **Determine if Heart Rate is within Range:**

If the heart rate satisfies the inequality (i.e., if 60 is less than or equal to 85, and 85 is less than or equal to 100), then it is within the acceptable range. Otherwise, it is not.

Example 4:

Determine the permissible values of x for the following inequality: $3x - 7 \geq 20$.

To solve the inequality $3x - 7 \geq 20$, you'll:

→ Isolate the Variable by adding 7 to both sides of the inequality to isolate the term containing x:
$$3x > 20 + 7$$
$$3x > 27$$

→ Simplify by dividing both sides by 3 to isolate x:
$$x > \frac{27}{3}$$
$$x > 9$$

→ Then you'll determine the permissible values and the permissible values of x are all real numbers greater than or equal to 9.

Therefore, the solution to the inequality $3x - 7 > 20$ is x is > 9.
(Action Steps)

Solving Inequalities

If you've gone through these examples, it is wise to practice these exercises on inequalities using the steps we explained earlier.

Exercise 1:

Solve the inequality and represent the solution on a number line:
a) $3x + 5 > 17$
b) $2 - 4x \leq -10$
c) $2x - 7 \leq 3x + 4$

Exercise 2:

a) Determine the permissible values of x for the following inequality: $3x - 7 > 20$.
b) A company requires employees to have at least 5 years of experience for a managerial position. Write an inequality to represent this requirement, and determine if a candidate with 8 years of experience meets the criterion.

➤ Word Problems Involving Algebraic Expressions

In this algebra concept, you'll encounter real-life situations that can be translated into or represented using algebraic expressions or equations. These problems require us to identify unknown quantities, set up appropriate expressions or equations based on the given information, and then solve for the unknowns using algebraic techniques.

Solving Word-Problems

These are the various steps thst will help you efficiently solve word-problems and we have simplified them for you.

The steps include:

- **Read the Problem Carefully:**

Understand the given information and what is being asked in the problem.

- **Identify the Unknowns:**

Determine the quantities that are unknown or need to be solved.

- **Translate the Information:**

Use variables to represent the unknown quantities and set up algebraic expressions or equations based on the given information.

- **Solve the Expressions or Equations:**

Use algebraic techniques to solve the expressions or equations for the unknown quantities.

- **Check the Solution:**

Verify that the solution makes sense in the context of problem and satisfies any given conditions.

Example 1:

A rectangular garden has a length that is 5 meters longer than its width. If the perimeter of the garden is 42 meters, find the dimensions of the garden.

Solution:

→ We have a rectangular garden with a known perimeter and need to find its dimensions.

→ To identify the unknowns, Let L represent the length of the garden and W represent the width.

→ After translating the information, we now know that the length is 5 meters longer than the width, so we can write the expression for the length as $L = W + 5$. The perimeter of a rectangle is given by $2L$

+ 2W\), so the perimeter of the garden is \(2(L + W)\), which is 42 meters.

→ To solve the equation we will be substituting \(L = W + 5\) into the expression for the perimeter, we get \(2((W + 5) + W) = 42\). Simplifying this equation gives us \(4W + 10 = 42\). Solving for \(W\), we find \(W = 8\). Substituting \(W = 8\) into \(L = W + 5\), we find \(L = 13\).

→ With a width of 8 meters and a length of 13 meters, the perimeter is indeed 42 meters. So, the solution correct.

This example illustrates how to solve a word problem involving algebraic expressions step by step.

Example 2:

A company charges a fixed monthly fee plus an additional charge for each service used. If a customer's bill for one month is $75 and they used 5 services, and each service costs $10, what is the company's fixed monthly fee?

Solution:

→ The problem provides information about a customer's bill, including the total amount paid and the number of services used.

→ We will identify the unknowns by letting \(F\) represent the fixed monthly fee.

→ Now translating the information, the total bill consists of the fixed monthly fee plus the additional charge for each service used. We can write the expression for the total bill as \(F + 5 \times 10\), since each service costs $10 and the customer used 5 services. According to the problem, the total bill is $75.

→ Setting up the equation to solve, we have \(F + 5 \times 10 = 75\). Simplifying, we get \(F + 50 = 75\). Subtracting 50 from both sides, we find \(F = 75 - 50 = 25\).

→ With a fixed monthly fee of $25 and 5 services used at $10 each, the total bill is indeed $75. So, the solution is right.

Solving Word-Problems Involving Algebraic Expressions

If you've gone through these examples, it is wise to practice these exercises on inequalities using the steps we explained earlier.

Exercise 1:

Solve these word-problems using the steps explained in the example.

a) A hospital's monthly expenses consist of a fixed administrative cost and a variable cost based on the number of patients treated. If the hospital's fixed administrative cost is $10,000 per month and it spends an additional $200 per patient treated, and the total monthly expenses amount to $20,000, how many patients does the hospital treat each month?

b) A nursing home schedules nursing shifts based on the number of residents in the facility. The monthly cost of nursing shifts includes a fixed cost for staffing plus an additional cost per resident. If the fixed staffing cost is $5,000 per month and the nursing home pays an additional $50 per resident, and the total monthly cost for nursing shifts is $10,000, how many residents are in the nursing home?

c) A medical clinic rents medical equipment on a monthly basis. The monthly rental cost consists of a fixed fee plus a variable fee based on the number of equipment units rented. If the clinic's fixed rental fee is $800 per month and it pays an additional $100 per equipment unit rented, and the total monthly rental cost amounts to $2,200, how many equipment units does the clinic rent each month?

➤ Graphing Linear Equations (Graphs)

Graphs provide a visual representation of data, equations, inequalities, functions, or relationships between variables. They help you understand how functions behaves in terms of changes and interacting with different values of x.

While, graphing linear equations involves plotting points on a coordinate plane to show the relationship between two variables. In linear equations, the relationship between the variables is represented by a straight line. For instance, imagine you have a math equation, like $y = 2x + 3$. This equation tells us how these two things, (x) and (y), are related using a straight line.

As a TEAS 7 student, you must learn to interpret graphs to extract information about key features such as points, lines, curves, and areas. You'll also need to learn it to identify peaks and valleys to determine seasonal patterns or trends and to also make predictions.

You will encounter graphs in questions related to temperature trends, population growth, and geometric shapes. For example, you might be asked to analyze a graph of temperature changes over time and to identify patterns or trends in weather data.

Graphing Linear Equations

These are the various steps for efficiently graphing linear equations and we have simplified them for you to understand easily.

The steps include:

- **Identify the Variables:**

In a linear equation, you typically have two variables, x and y.

- **Choose Values for x:**

Pick some values for x to create a table of ordered pairs. These values can be any numbers you like, but it's often helpful to choose numbers that are easy to work with. For example, we might choose $x = 0$, $x = 1$, $x = 2$, and so on.

- **Find the Corresponding y Values:**

Substitute each value of x into the equation to find the corresponding y values.

- **Plot the Points:**

Plot the ordered pairs (x, y) on the coordinate plane.

- **Draw the Line:**

Connect the points with a straight line to represent the graph of the equation.

Example 1:

Let's graph the linear equation $y = 2x + 3$.

- → In this equation, x and y are the variables that we'll pick.
- → We can choose a few values for x, such as $x = -2$, $x = 0$, and $x = 2$.
- → Once we have our x values, we use the equation to figure out what y is for each value of x we picked. To do this, we will substitute each value of x into the equation to find the corresponding y values:
  - For $x = -2$: $y = 2(-2) + 3 = -4 + 3 = -1$
  - For $x = 0$: $y = 2(0) + 3 = 0 + 3 = 3$
  - For $x = 2$: $y = 2(2) + 3 = 4 + 3 = 7$
- → We'll plot the ordered pairs (-2, -1), (0, 3), and (2, 7) on the coordinate plane.
- → Then we'll connect the points with a straight line. This line represents the relationship between x and y described by the equation.

So, the graph of the linear equation $y = 2x + 3$ will be a straight line passing through the points (-2, -1), (0, 3), and (2, 7).

This example demonstrates how you can graph a linear equation by plotting the points and connecting them with a line.

Example 2:

Let's consider the linear equation $(y = 2x + 3)$ and graph it:

→ The equation $(y = 2x + 3)$ represents a linear relationship between (x) and (y), where (2) is the slope of the line, and (3) is the y-intercept.

→ To graph the equation, we start by plotting points. We can choose any values for (x) and then calculate the corresponding values for (y) using the equation. Let's choose three values for (x): -2, 0, and 2.

   - When $(x = -2)$, $(y = 2(-2) + 3 = -4 + 3 = -1)$. So, the point (-2, -1) is on the line.

   - When $(x = 0)$, $(y = 2(0) + 3 = 0 + 3 = 3)$. So, the point (0, 3) is on the line.

   - When $(x = 2)$, $(y = 2(2) + 3 = 4 + 3 = 7)$. So, the point (2, 7) is on the line.

→ Now, plot the points (-2, -1), (0, 3), and (2, 7) on the coordinate plane.

→ Once the points are plotted, draw a straight line passing through these points. Since the equation represents a linear relationship, the line will be straight.

→ The graph of the linear equation $(y = 2x + 3)$ is a straight line with a slope of (2) and a y-intercept of (3).

This means that for every unit increase in (x), (y) increases by (2), and the line crosses the y-axis at the point (0, 3).

Example 3:

Graphical Linear Equations Involving World Problems:

A medical clinic tracks its monthly expenses for staffing and equipment maintenance. The clinic's monthly staffing expenses are $3000, and its monthly equipment maintenance expenses are $2000. Write a linear equation to represent the clinic's total monthly expenses T in dollars based on the number of staff members S employed. Then, graph the equation to visualize the relationship between total monthly expenses and staffing levels.

Solution:

→ **Understanding the Problem:**
     - The problem states that the medical clinic has monthly staffing expenses of $3000 and monthly equipment maintenance expenses of $2000.
     - You'll need to represent the total monthly expenses T in dollars based on the number of staff members S employed using a linear equation.
     - Afterward, you'll'll graph the equation to visualize the relationship between total monthly expenses and staffing levels.

→ **Writing the Linear Equation:**
     - You'll denote T as the total monthly expenses in dollars and S as the number of staff members employed.
     - The total monthly expenses consist of the staffing expenses ($3000) and the equipment maintenance expenses ($2000).
     - So, the linear equation representing the total monthly expenses is: $T = 3000 + 2000S$.

→ **Plotting Points and Graphing the Equation:**
     - To graph the equation, you can choose several values for S and calculate the corresponding values for T using the equation.
     - So let's choose three values for S: 0, 5, and 10 staff members.
     - When $S = 0$, $T = 3000 + 2000(0) = 3000$. So, the point (0, 3000) is on the line.

- When $S = 5$, $T = 3000 + 2000(5) = 3000 + 10000 = 13000$.
  So, the point (5, 13000) is on the line.
- When $S = 10$, $T = 3000 + 2000(10) = 3000 + 20000 = 23000$.
So, the point (10, 23000) is on the line.

→ Now, plot these points on the coordinate plane and draw a straight line passing through them.

→ **Interpreting the Graph:**
- The graph of the linear equation $T = 3000 + 2000S$ is a straight line with a positive slope, indicating that as the number of staff members employed increases, the total monthly expenses also increase linearly.

(Action Steps)
Graphing Linear Equations

If you've gone through these examples, it is wise to practice these exercises on inequalities using the steps we explained earlier.

Exercise 1:

Consider the linear equation $y = -2x + 5$.

a) Plot the graph of this equation, and then identify two points on the graph.

b) A medical research facility has fixed monthly expenses of $10,000 and additional expenses of $100 per hour for equipment usage. Write a linear equation to represent the facility's total monthly expenses T based on the number of hours of equipment usage H, and then graph the equation to visualize the relationship between total monthly expenses and equipment usage hours.

Data Interpretation:
How To Understand and Analyze Data

Data interpretation refers to the process of analyzing, understanding, and making sense of data presented in various forms such as tables, charts, graphs, or textual formats.

It's about figuring out what the data is telling you, such as finding patterns, trends, or relationship, extracting meaningful insights, so that you can use it in making decisions or learning more about a topic.

This process often involves looking at the data carefully, critically thinking about what it means, and interpreting the information accurately and effectively, through your statistical analysis skills. Data Interpretation is very important in areas like science, business, and healthcare because it aids in making better decisions based on the information gotten.

In the context of the TEAS 7 examination, this skill is very important because it's a part of the exam and your ability to understand and analyze information presented in different ways, like tables, charts, graphs, and passages will be tested. You'll be asked to interpret data to answer questions about scientific experiments or make decisions based on patient data in healthcare scenarios. So, being good at interpreting data helps them do well on the exam.

Now let's move on to the techniques that will help you understand and analyze data in formats like tables, charts and graphs perfectly.

Techniques For Understanding And Analyzing Data

These techniques will help you understand and analyze data in a simple way and you'll be able to uncover insights, trends, patterns, anomalies, and relationships that can inform your decision-making, solve problems, or support research objectives. So you can easily understand and analyze any data presented to you by:

➤ Reviewing the Data:

First, you'll need to see what kind of information you have. This means you'll check the dataset to understand its structure, contents, and context.

You'll also need to know what type of data you're dealing with (e.g., numerical, categorical), how it's organized, where it came from or represents. Understanding the data's origin and any potential biases or limitations is essential for interpreting the results accurately.

➤ Identifying Patterns:

You'll need to look for recurring trends, relationships, or patterns in the data. This could be things like numbers going up (increasing) or down over time (decreasing), trends, or groups of similar data. Most visualization techniques, such as line graphs, scatter plots, or histograms, can help reveal these patterns to you more effectively than examining raw numbers alone

➤ Summarizing Data:

This means using numbers to describe the main things about the data. By numbers, were talking about using descriptive statistics such as mean, median, mode, and range to summarize the central tendency, most common value, and variability of the data. Summarizing the data in this way can help you understand its distribution, characteristics, and also make it easier for you to interpret and compare.

➤ Visualizing Data:

Next, you'll create visual representations of the data using graphs, charts, or tables to make it easier for you to identify patterns and trends rather than looking at raw numbers alone. You can use visualization methods such as bar charts, pie charts, line graphs, and heat maps. However, choosing the right visualization depends on the type of data and the insights you're trying to convey.

➢ Comparing Data:

Comparing data will help you how different parts of the data are similar, different, or have changed over time. Your data comparison could be from different groups, people, locations, or time periods. Statistical tests, such as t-tests or chi-square tests, can also help you determine whether your observed differences are statistically significant.

➢ Using Statistical Analysis:

You can use more statistical methods to analyze the data more rigorously, such as hypothesis testing to evaluate relationships between variables, regression analysis to model relationships between variables, or analysis of variance (ANOVA) to compare means across multiple groups.

Also, statistical software packages like R, Python with libraries like NumPy and pandas, or specialized software such as SPSS or SAS, are commonly used for these analyses. So you can try them out too

➢ Data Mining:

You'll need to use this data mining technique to uncover hidden patterns or insights because there are things in the data that may not be obvious at first. Techniques like clustering, classification, and association rule mining can reveal the relationships and dependencies within the data that may not be immediately apparent. Some data mining algorithms, such as k-means clustering or decision trees, can also automatically identify patterns and structures in the data.

➢ Interpreting Results:

Finally, you need to think about what the data is telling you. Draw meaningful conclusions and make informed decisions based on the analysis of the data. You'll do this when you consider the context of the data, including any relevant background information or domain knowledge. It's also essential that you acknowledge any limitations or biases present in the data and consider if there are other reasons for these observed patterns.

Applying these techniques as a TEAS 7 student will make you gain a deeper understanding of the data and use it to inform your decision-making, problem-solving, and research in various fields effectively.

Chapter 5:

Understanding Science

Science plays a crucial role in our everyday life. It influences everything. From the functioning of the human body to medical treatments and technologies that will make us hale and hearty. So whether you're aspiring to become a nurse, doctor, or allied healthcare professional, having a solid understanding of these scientific principles is indispensible.

In this chapter, we will explore the fundamental principles of science as well as focus more on some core concepts in anatomy, physiology, chemistry, and biology. These core concepts serve as the foundation for understanding more complex topics within anatomy, physiology, chemistry, and biology. So mastery of these concepts is crucial for your success in the science section of your TEAS 7 examination and your healthcare career.

This chapter will also cover the basic ideas in anatomy (how our bodies are built), physiology (how our bodies function), chemistry (how substances interact), and biology (how living things work). We'll keep things simple but cover everything you need to know.

We'll also talk about how to apply scientific knowledge effectively in real life. This means how you can think critically about scientific ideas and solve problems like a healthcare professional or scientist.

To reinforce your learning, we have included action steps such as science exercises focused on these science topics. These interactive exercises will allow you to assess your understanding, identify areas for improvement, and solidify your knowledge in preparation for the exam.

So, let's get started!

What is Science and its Relevance to the TEAS 7 Exam:

Science is all about studying the natural world through experiments, observations, and analysis. It covers subjects like anatomy, biology, chemistry, physics, and earth sciences.

In the healthcare world, science is like the building blocks that help us understand how our bodies work, what makes us sick, and how we can get better. The healthcare workers use science to diagnose illnesses, create treatment plans, and make sure patients stay healthy. For example, knowing about anatomy helps doctors understand where our organs are and how they work, while biology helps them understand why diseases happen.

When it comes to the TEAS 7 exam, knowing science is super important, especially for the Science section. Especially as this part of the test evaluates your knowledge and comprehension of the fundamental scientific concepts, principles, and processes relevant to healthcare professions. Now, we move on to discuss the core concepts in anatomy, biology, physics, and chemistry so that you can be well grounded and ready for the science section of the TEAS 7 exam.

➢ **Anatomy**

Anatomy is all about understanding how our bodies are built. It's like knowing how all the pieces fit together inside us, from our bones to our organs and everything in between.

It is the branch of science that deals with the study of the structure and organization of living organisms and their parts. It explores the arrangement of cells, tissues, organs, and organ systems within the body, as well as their relationships to one another. Anatomy provides a detailed understanding of the body's physical makeup, including the size, shape, location, and the function of its various components.

The Importance of Anatomy in Healthcare:

Anatomy plays an important role in healthcare for several reasons:

- **It Helps with Diagnosis and Treatment:**

Healthcare professionals, such as physicians, surgeons, nurses, and allied health professionals, rely on anatomical knowledge to diagnose medical conditions accurately and develop effective treatment plans. Understanding how different parts of our bodies are supposed to look like helps them figure out when something's wrong. For example, Abnormalities like swelling in the body may indicate disease or injury.

- **It Guides Surgeries:**

Surgeons rely on anatomy to know exactly where to cut and what to avoid during surgical operations. Knowledge of anatomical landmarks, structures, and relationships helps them do their job safely effectively as well as minimizes the risk of complications during procedures.

- **It Aids in Patient Care and Management:**

Nurses and other healthcare workers use their knowledge of anatomy to assess patients, monitor their health status, and provide appropriate care. For example, understanding the anatomy of the cardiovascular system helps clinicians assess heart function, diagnose cardiac conditions, and manage cardiovascular diseases.

- **It Helps in interpreting Medical Images:**

When we get X-rays or scans, doctors use anatomy to understand what they're seeing. It helps them spot any abnormality and accurately decide on the best treatment.

- **It Drives Medical Research:**

Anatomy serves as the foundation for biomedical research and innovation in healthcare. Scientists and researchers study the anatomy of the human body to advance medical knowledge, develop new treatments, and improve healthcare technologies. It also helps in designing medical devices, developing pharmaceuticals, and conducting clinical trials.

- **It Helps Patients Understand:**

Doctors use anatomy to explain what is going on in patients bodies and how they can better take care of their bodies in a way that they can understand. Educating patients about their body also helps them make informed decisions and actively participate in care.

Now, let's head on to the structure and functions of the human body.

The Structure and Function of the Human Body

The structure of anatomy refers to the arrangement and organization of the various components within the human body. This includes bones, muscles, organs, tissues, and cells, as well as their spatial relationships and connections. All these will be discussed as you read on.

➢ Skeleton (Bones):

The skeleton is like the frame of a house. It's made up of bones that structure, support, and protect our organs and body. The skeletal system is made up of 206 bones in adults, although this number can vary slightly between individuals.

The bones in the human body vary in size, shape, and density, with each serving specific functions. They are comprised of cells embedded in a matrix of collagen fibers and mineral deposits, primarily calcium and phosphate which provides them with strength and flexibility. They are also complex organs made up of various tissues such as bone tissue, cartilage, blood vessels, nerves, and connective tissues.

- **Types of Bones:**

Bones are classified into five main categories based on their shape: long bones, short bones, flat bones, irregular bones, and sesamoid bones. Each type serves specific functions in the body.

→ **Long Bones:** These bones are longer than there width and typically have a shaft (diaphysis) and two ends (epiphyses). Examples include our leg bones; femur, humerus, radius, and ulna.

→ **Short Bones:** These bones are roughly cube-shaped and give support and stability with limited movement to our wrists and ankles. Examples include the carpals in the wrist and tarsals in the ankle.

→ **Flat Bones:** These bones are thin and flattened, often with a curved shape. They provide protection for underlying organs and serve as attachment sites for muscles. Examples include the shoulder blades, skull bones (parietal, frontal), ribs, scapulae, and sternum.

→ **Irregular Bones:** Irregular bones have complex shapes and do not fit into the categories of long, short, or flat bones. They just have unique shapes. Examples include the vertebrae (backbones), facial bones (mandible, maxilla), and pelvic bones.

→ **Sesamoid Bones:** Sesamoid bones are small, round bones embedded within tendons (the tissues that connect muscles to bones), where they provide protection and improve mechanical efficiency. The patella (kneecap) is the largest sesamoid bone in the body.

- **The Microscopic Structure**

At the microscopic level, bones are composed of a dense outer layer called compact bone, which provides strength and protection.

→ Within compact bone are numerous channels called Haversian canals, which contain blood vessels, lymphatic vessels, and nerves.

→ Surrounding the Haversian canals are concentric layers of bone matrix called lamellae, which contain mineral salts (mainly hydroxyapatite) and collagen fibers.

→ Embedded within the bone matrix are osteocytes, mature bone cells, which maintain bone tissue and play a role in mineral homeostasis.

→ The osteocytes communicate with each other and with the blood supply through tiny channels called canaliculi, allowing for the exchange of nutrients and waste products.

- **Bone Development and Growth:** *How do bones develop?*

Bones develop through a process called ossification, which begins during embryonic development and continues throughout childhood and adolescence.

Just incase you do not know, Ossification occurs through two main processes: intramembranous ossification, where bone forms directly within mesenchymal tissue, and endochondral ossification, where bone forms within a cartilage model.

Throughout our lives, bones undergo constant remodeling, a process of resorption (removal of old bone tissue) by osteoclasts and deposition (formation of new bone tissue) by osteoblasts. This remodeling process helps them maintain bone strength, repair micro damage, and regulate mineral homeostasis.

- **Functions of The Bone:**

The bones perform various fuctions such as:

→ **Support:** Bones provide a structure that supports the body's soft tissues, muscles, and organs, allowing us to stand, move, and maintain our posture. It also gives the body shape and rigidity.

→ **Protection:** Bones protect vital organs such as the brain, heart, lungs, and spinal cord from mechanical injury and trauma. For example, the skull protects the brain, the rib cage protects the heart and lungs, and the vertebrae protect the spinal cord.

→ **Movement:** Bones, along with muscles, joints, and ligaments, form the musculoskeletal system and thet enable movement and locomotion. Muscles attach to bones via tendons and exert forces to produce movement.

→ **Mineral Storage:** Bones serve as a reservoir for minerals such as calcium, phosphorus, and magnesium. These minerals are essential for various metabolic processes and physiological functions such as muscle contraction, nerve conduction, and blood clotting.

→ **Blood Cell Formation:** Certain bones, particularly the flat bones of the skull, ribs, sternum, and pelvis, contain red bone marrow, where hematopoiesis occurs. Hematopoiesis is the process of producing blood cells like erythrocytes (red blood cells), leukocytes (white blood cells), and platelets.

➢ **Muscles**

Muscles are vital components of the human body, responsible for movement, stability, and maintaining posture. They are like rubber bands in our body because they are composed of special tissues capable of stretching, contracting and relaxing in response to nerve signals.

Each muscle consists of muscle fibers arranged in bundles and these fibers are made up of smaller units called myofibrils, containing proteins called actin and myosin, responsible for muscle contraction.

Muscles attach to the bones via tough, fibrous tissues called tendons. So, when they contract, they pull on these tendons, which in turn pull on the bones and makes our body parts move. For example, when we bend our arm, the muscles in our arm contract, pulling on the bones in our arm and causing it to bend.

• **Types of Muscles**

The various types of muscles found in the human body include:

→ **Skeletal Muscles:** These are the muscles attached to bones and are under voluntary control; we can control them with our brains. When we decide to move our arms or legs, our brain sends signals to these muscles to make them work. Skeletal muscles enable voluntary movements such as walking, lifting, and facial expressions.

→ **Smooth Muscles:** These muscles are found in the walls of hollow organs such as the stomach, intestines, and blood vessels, smooth muscles are involuntary; they work without us thinking about them and they regulate various internal processes like digestion and blood flow.

→ **Cardiac Muscles:** This special muscle is only in our heart. The cardiac muscle is involuntary and responsible for the rhythmic contractions that pump blood in the heart and throughout the body.

- **Functions of Muscles**

The functions of the muscles in the body include:

→ Muscles facilitate movement by generating force when they contract. This force pulls on the bones, causing them to move around joints. It enable actions such as walking, lifting, and facial expressions.

→ They contribute to maintaining your body posture and stability by counteracting the force of gravity and supporting your body's weight.

→ Muscles are also involved in essential bodily functions such as breathing, circulation, and digestion, through the coordinated contractions of smooth and cardiac muscle tissue.

➢ **Organs**

Organs are like the different rooms in a house with specific shapes and functions. They are vital anatomical structures composed of different tissues that work together as a team to perform specific functions necessary for the body's survival and optimal health. Examples of organs in the human body include the heart, lungs, liver, kidneys, brain, and stomach, among others.

Each organ in the body has a unique structure that reflects its function, and they are made up of different tissues that help them do their jobs well. For example, the heart which is made up of the cardiac muscle tissue pumps blood. The liver contains the hepatocytes cell responsible for metabolizing toxins and synthesizing proteins. The lungs make us breathe and the stomach digests food.

The organs in the human body play critical roles in maintaining homeostasis, which refers to the body's ability to regulate internal conditions such as temperature, pH, and nutrient levels within narrow ranges.

They also interact with each other and with other systems in the body through complex networks of nerves, blood vessels, and hormones to coordinate physiological processes and respond to external stimuli.

Understanding the structure and function of organs is very important in healthcare professions like medicine and nursing because the practitioners rely on this knowledge to diagnose diseases, develop treatment plans, and provide care to patients effectively.

Additionally, research in anatomy contributes to advancements in medical technologies, surgical techniques, and therapeutic interventions which are aimed at improving the patients outcomes and enhancing their overall health and well-being.

- **Organs and Their Functions**

Here is a simple explanation of some key organs and their functions:

→ **Heart:** The heart is a muscular organ located in the chest cavity, slightly to the left. It consists of four chambers: two atria (upper chambers) and two ventricles (lower chambers).

It is composed of specialized cardiac muscle tissue and it's primary function is to pump blood throughout the body, deliver oxygen and nutrients to cells and remove waste products from the body.

The atria receive blood from the body and lungs, while the ventricles pump blood out to the body and lungs, respectively.

→ **Lungs:** The lungs are paired organs situated in the chest cavity, protected by the rib cage. Each lung is divided into lobes and contains bronchial tubes, alveoli (air sacs), and blood vessels. Also, the lung tissue is made up of elastic and spongy tissue.

The primary function of the lung is to facilitate the exchange of oxygen and carbon dioxide during breathing. Oxygen from inhaled air diffuses into the bloodstream through the alveoli, while carbon dioxide is expelled from the body during exhalation. This just means that it help us breathe by taking in oxygen from the air and getting rid of carbon dioxide.

→ **Liver:** The liver is the largest internal organ located in the upper right abdomen. It has a unique lobular structure and is made up of hepatocytes (liver cells) organized into lobules. Blood vessels and bile ducts traverse the liver tissue.

The liver performs numerous vital functions, including detoxification of harmful substances, metabolism of nutrients and drugs, production of bile for digestion, storage of glycogen, and synthesis of proteins essential for blood clotting and immune function. This simply means that it helps clean our blood, digest food, and store energy.

→ **Kidneys:** The kidneys are bean-shaped organs located in the abdominal cavity, one on each side of the spine. They are made up of renal cortex, medulla, and renal pelvis.

Each kidney consists of millions of nephrons, which are the functional units responsible for filtering blood and producing urine. The functions of the kidneys is to regulate fluid balance, electrolyte levels, and acid-base balance in the body by filtering waste products, excess ions, and water from the bloodstream to form urine.

They also play a crucial role in blood pressure regulation and hormone production.

→ **Brain:** The brain is the command center of the nervous system and it is protected by the skull. It comprises various regions, including the cerebrum, cerebellum, and brainstem, each with distinct structures and functions.

Also, it contains neurons (nerve cells) and glial cells. The brain coordinates sensory perception, motor control, cognition, emotion, and involuntary bodily functions.

It processes and interprets information received from the senses, controls movement, stores memories, and regulates basic physiological processes like heartbeat and breathing. In summary, it controls everything we do, like thinking, moving, and feeling.

➤ Nervous System

The nervous system is like the body's electrical wiring sending signals and messages between different parts of the body and the brain; which allows us to move, think, feel, and respond to changes in our surroundings.

The nervous system is a complex network of nerves and cells that transmit signals between different parts of the body. It coordinates and controls bodily functions and responses to stimuli, allowing organisms to interact with their environment and maintain homeostasis.

It is made up of the brain, spinal cord, and nerves, and it is organized into the central nervous system (CNS) and peripheral nervous system (PNS).

- **Parts of The Nervous System**

The nervous system is divided into two main parts:

→ **Central Nervous System (CNS):**
The central nervous system consists of the brain and spinal cord. It serves as the main processing center for all incoming and outgoing signals.

The brain is divided into several parts including the cerebrum (for thinking and memory), cerebellum (for balance and coordination), and brainstem (for basic functions like breathing and heartbeat).

Each is responsible for specific functions such as cognition, movement, and sensory perception. The brain interprets sensory information, processes thoughts and emotions, and sends out commands to the rest of the body.

While, the spinal cord is a long, tubular structure encased within the spinal column (vertebrae) and serves as a conduit for nerve signals between the brain and the rest of the body. It acts as a relay between the brain and the peripheral nervous system, transmitting signals to and from the body.

→ **Peripheral Nervous System (PNS):**

The peripheral nervous system includes all the nerves outside the brain and spinal cord. It includes cranial nerves (connected to the brain) and spinal nerves (connected to the spinal cord). The PNS helps with things like moving our muscles and feeling things like pain or touch.

The Peripheral Nervous System (PNS) is further divided into the somatic nervous system and the autonomic nervous system. The somatic nervous system controls voluntary movements and sensory input from the body's surface, such as touch, temperature, and pain. The sensory nerves sends signals to the brain while the motor nerves controls the muscles.

The autonomic nervous system regulates involuntary functions like heart rate, digestion, and breathing. It is further subdivided into the sympathetic and parasympathetic nervous systems, which work together to maintain internal balance (homeostasis) by responding to changes in the external and internal environment.

➤ **Digestive System**

The digestive system is a complex network of organs and processes responsible for breaking down food into nutrients that the body can absorb and utilize for energy, growth, and repair.

It consists of several organs, each with specific functions that contribute to the overall process of ingestion, digestion, absorption, and elimination of food and waste products in the body.

The digestive system consists of the gastrointestinal tract (mouth, esophagus, stomach, small intestine, large intestine) and accessory organs (liver, gallbladder, pancreas).

Its primary function is to break down food into nutrients (e.g., carbohydrates, proteins, fats) that can be absorbed and utilized by the body. Also, the mechanical and chemical processes in the digestive tract facilitate digestion and absorption, while the accessory organs secrete enzymes and bile to aid in nutrient breakdown and absorption. The digestive system also eliminates indigestible waste as feces.

- **Components of The Digestive System**

Here is a simple breakdown of the digestive system:

→ **Mouth:** This is where digestion begins. It is the entry point of the digestive system and it begins the process of digestion by mechanically breaking down food through chewing and mixing it with saliva.

The saliva is produced by the salivary glands which contains enzymes, such as amylase, responsible for starting the chemical breakdown of carbohydrates and it's digestion.

For example, after chewing, the saliva enzymes break down carbohydrates like bread and pasta into simpler sugars. In simple terms: Your teeth chew food into smaller pieces, and your saliva helps break it down.

→ **Esophagus:** The esophagus is a muscular tube that connects the mouth to the stomach. It transports chewed food from the mouth to the stomach through a series of coordinated contractions known as peristalsis.

So, when you swallow food, the muscles in your esophagus squeeze and push the food down toward your stomach. The primary function of the esophagus is to facilitate the movement of food bolus from the oral cavity to the stomach for further digestion.

Also, the esophageal sphincter at the bottom of the esophagus prevents food from refluxing back into the mouth.

→ **Stomach:** The stomach is a hollow, muscular organ located in the upper abdomen. It serves as a storage reservoir for food and further breaks down food mechanically through churning and mixes it with gastric juices containing hydrochloric acid and digestive enzymes like pepsin.

These enzymes break down proteins into smaller peptides, initiating protein digestion. In simple terms: The stomach is like a mixing bowl. It churns the food and mixes it with stomach juices that help break it down further.

→ **Small Intestine:** The small intestine is the longest segment of the digestive tract and is where most of the digestion and nutrient absorption take place. It is divided into three regions: the duodenum, jejunum, and ileum.

Enzymes from the pancreas and bile from the liver help break down carbohydrates, proteins, and fats into their component molecules, which are then absorbed into the bloodstream through the intestinal lining.

→ **Large Intestine (Colon):** The large intestine, or colon, follows the small intestine and is responsible for reabsorbing water and electrolytes from undigested food particles.

It also houses a diverse population of beneficial bacteria known as the gut microbiota,which plays a crucial role in aiding fermentation, production of certain vitamins, and maintenance of gut health. In simple terms: Your body absorbs water from the leftovers and turns them into solid waste (poop).

→ **Rectum and Anus:** The rectum and anus form the final portion of the digestive tract and they are responsible for the elimination of indigestible waste material in form of feces.

Muscular contractions in the colon propel fecal matter into the rectum, where it is stored until defecation occurs through the relaxation of anal sphincter muscles.

➢ **Respiratory System**

The respiratory system is a critical component of human anatomy that is made up of complex network of organs and tissues responsible for the exchange of gases between the body and the environment.

Not just that, the respiratory system also helps regulate blood pH and plays a role in vocalization and olfaction. The respiratory system comprises the airways (nose, pharynx, larynx, trachea, bronchi, bronchioles) and lungs.

It's primary function is to facilitate the intake of oxygen and the removal of carbon dioxide through inhalation and exhalation. The inhalation brings air into the lungs where oxygen diffuses into the bloodstream, and carbon dioxide is expelled during exhalation.

These are essential processes needed for cellular respiration and overall metabolic function.

In simple terms: The respiratory system is all about breathing, getting oxygen into our body, and getting rid of carbon dioxide as a waste product.

• **Parts of The Respiratory System**

Now, let's explain the different parts of the respiratory system that work together to help us breathe and stay alive.

→ **Nose and Mouth:** The nose and mouth are the body's entry points for air. This of course is where the respiratory process begins. These entry points filter, warm, and humidify the air before it reaches the lower respiratory tract. The nasal passages are lined with mucous membranes and tiny hair-like structures called cilia, which trap foreign particles and pathogens in a way that prevents them from entering the lungs.

→ **Pharynx and Larynx (Throat and Voice Box):** After passing through the nose or mouth, air travels through the pharynx (throat), a common passageway for both air and food. The larynx or voice box, which is located below the pharynx houses the vocal cords in charge of producing speech and preventing food and liquids from entering the airway during swallowing.

→ **Trachea (Windpipe):** The trachea is like a straw for breathing. It is a rigid, tubular structure composed of cartilage rings that connect the larynx to the bronchi. It serves as a conduit for air to travel from the upper respiratory tract to the lungs. The trachea is lined with mucous membranes and cilia, which continue the process of filtering and humidifying the air.

→ **Bronchial Tubes (Bronchi and Bronchioles):** These are the airways that carry air from the trachea into the lungs. The trachea branches into two main bronchi, one leading to each lung. Within the lungs, the bronchi is further divide into smaller airways called bronchioles. These airways ensure the passage of oxygen-rich air to the alveoli and also the removes carbon dioxide-laden air. The bronchial tubes are surrounded by smooth muscle that allow constriction and dilation to regulate airflow.

→ **Lungs:** The lungs situated within the thoracic cavity, are the primary organs of respiration. They are responsible for the exchange of gases between the air and the bloodstream. Each lung is enclosed within a pleural membrane and divided into lobes (three on the right and two on the left). Now, inside these lungs are smaller tubes called bronchi and bronchioles which function is to help carry air to the different body parts.

→ **Alveoli (Air Sacs):** These are tiny, microscopic air sacs located at the end of the bronchial tree (the lungs), These thin-walled structures provide an extensive surface area for the exchange of oxygen and carbon dioxide to occur. They are like little balloons where oxygen from the air we breathe in passes through the walls of the alveoli and into our bloodstream, while carbon dioxide moves from the blood into the alveoli to be breathed out.

→ **Diaphragm and Respiratory Muscles:** The diaphragm is the primary muscle involved in breathing. It separates the thoracic cavity (containing the lungs and heart) from the abdominal cavity. When we breathe in, the diaphragm contracts and moves downward, creating more space in our chest for the lungs to expand and fill with air.

When we breathe out, the diaphragm relaxes and moves back up, pushing the air out of our lungs. There are other respiratory muscles like the intercostal muscles between the ribs that contribute to the breathing process.

→ **Rib Cage:** The rib cage is made up of ribs, sternum, and thoracic vertebrae which surrounds and safeguards your lungs and other organs of the respiratory system. They are also connected to the spine in the back and the breastbone in the front.

Knowing the respiratory system and keeping yours and that of other patients healthy is important for the body's overall well-being. It is also important to avoid things like smoking or breathing in harmful chemicals that can damage the lungs and make it harder to breathe.

Anatomical Terminology and Body Planes

Anatomical terminology is a standardized language used by healthcare professionals to describe the structures, positions, and relationships of the human body.

It provides precise terms to accurately communicate information about different features of the human body and about the direction of movements and the orientation of imaging scans or surgical incisions.

This standardized language ensures accurate descriptions, diagnoses, and treatments, that ultimately improves the patient care and safety.

In summary, anatomical terminology and body planes serve as the foundation for effective communication and understanding within the healthcare field. It facilitates accurate descriptions of the human body's complex structures and functions.

- **Directional Terms**
  → **Anterior and Posterior:** Anterior refers to the front or forward-facing aspect of the body, while posterior refers to the back or rear-facing aspect. For instance, the eyes are anterior to the brain.
  → **Superior and Inferior:** Superior indicates a higher position or location above another structure, whereas inferior indicates a lower position or location below another structure. For example, the head is superior to the neck.
  → **Medial and Lateral:** The medial describes a position closer to the midline or center of the body, while lateral describes a position farther away from the midline. The nose is medial to the ears.
  → **Proximal and Distal:** Proximal denotes a position closer to the point of origin or attachment, while distal denotes a position farther away from the point of origin or attachment. For instance, the elbow is proximal to the wrist.
  → **Superficial and Deep:** Superficial refers to a position closer to the surface of the body, whereas deep refers to a position deeper within the body or further away from the surface.

→ **Central and Peripheral:** Central describes structures located near the center of an organ or system, while peripheral describes structures located towards the outer edges or away from the center.

- **Body Planes**

Body planes are imaginary flat surfaces used to visualize and dissect the body for anatomical study. They help describe the orientation and spatial relationships of anatomical structures. The three primary body planes are:

→ **Sagittal Plane:** The sagittal plane divides the body into right and left halves, running longitudinally from front to back. A mid-sagittal plane divides the body into equal right and left halves, while a parasagittal plane divides the body into unequal right and left portions.

→ **Frontal Plane:** Also known as the coronal plane, this plane divides the body into anterior (front) and posterior (back) portions, running longitudinally from side to side.

→ **Transverse Plane:** This plane divides the body into upper (superior) and lower (inferior) portions, running horizontally from side to side. It is perpendicular to both the sagittal and frontal planes.

Illustrations of various anatomical concepts

Example 1: *Anatomical Terminology*

Scenario: A medical student is studying the anatomy of the human heart.

Explanation: The student identifies the anterior surface of the heart, referring to the side facing forward in the body. They also identify the posterior surface, which faces backward.

Additionally, they describe the apex of the heart, referring to the pointed tip, and the base, which is the broader superior portion. By using anatomical terminology, the student accurately communicates the location and orientation of different heart structures.

Example 2: *Body Planes*

Scenario: A surgical team is preparing for an appendectomy procedure.

Explanation: The surgeon discusses the surgical approach with the team, referring to specific body planes to ensure precision and accuracy during the procedure. They plan to make an incision along the midline of the body, known as the median or midsagittal plane, to access the appendix.

By understanding body planes, the surgical team can visualize the internal structures in relation to the incision site and navigate safely to the target area. This will minimize any risk and complication.

> ➤ **Physiology**

Physiology is the branch of biology that focuses on understandimg how living organisms function at various levels, from the molecular and cellular levels to the whole organism level.

It involves understanding the mechanisms and processes enabling organisms to carry out vital functions in the body that maintain life and health, such as respiration, circulation, digestion, metabolism, and reproduction.

Physiology seeks to explain how different organ systems work together to maintain homeostasis, respond to stimuli, and adapt to changes in the internal and external environment. It investigates various systems of the body, such as the nervous system, cardiovascular system, respiratory system, digestive system, and endocrine system, among others.

It also examines how these systems work individually and in coordination with each other to carry out vital functions necessary for survival. For example, in the cardiovascular system, physiology explores how the heart pumps blood through the body, how blood vessels regulate blood pressure, and how blood transports nutrients, oxygen, and waste products.

In the respiratory system, physiology examines the process of breathing, gas exchange in the lungs, and the regulation of respiratory rate to maintain proper oxygen levels in the body.

Overall, physiology provides insights into the complex mechanisms that allow organisms to respond to changes in their environment, maintain internal balance (homeostasis), and adapt to various physiological challenges. It is fundamental to understanding health and disease and plays a crucial role in fields such as medicine, sports science, and biomedical research.

The knowledge of key physiological concepts is essential for the success of you, a TEAS 7 exam candidate and also for pursuing a career in healthcare where understanding how the body functions is fundamental.

Importance of Physiology to The Healthcare World

- **Gives Understanding of The Human Body Functions:**

Physiology provides you with insights into how the body's organs, tissues, and cells function under normal conditions.

This is through the study of physiological processes such as digestion, respiration, circulation, and nervous system function, healthcare professionals can better understand how the body maintains homeostasis and responds to internal and external stimuli. This knowledge is essential for diagnosing and treating diseases, as deviations from normal physiological functions often indicate underlying health issues.

- **Improves Medical Diagnostics and Treatment:**

Physiology serves as the basis for medical diagnostics and treatment strategies. Healthcare practitioners use physiological principles to interpret clinical findings, assess patient health, and formulate treatment plans.

For example, understanding cardiovascular physiology helps cardiologists diagnose and manage heart conditions, while knowledge of respiratory physiology guides pulmonologists in treating respiratory disorders. When physiological concepts are applied in clinical practice, healthcare professionals can optimize patient care and outcomes.

- **Advances Medical Research and Innovation:**

Physiology drives medical research and innovation by uncovering the underlying mechanisms of health and disease. When researchers explore physiological processes at the molecular, cellular, tissue, organ, and systemic levels to identify disease pathways, they develop new therapies and improve medical technologies.

For instance, understanding the physiological basis of cancer has led to the development of targeted therapies and immunotherapies that selectively target cancer cells while minimizing damage to healthy tissues. By increasing the knowledge of physiology, researchers can address complex health challenges and pave the way for more medical breakthroughs.

Key Concepts Under Physiology

There are different types of physiology containing important physiological concepts and principles that are essential for understanding how your body functions and responds to different stimuli. Here, two key concepts will be discussed interestingly, to give you a thorough understanding that will aid the success of your TEAS 7 examination.

➢ Human Physiology

Human physiology is the study of how the human body works. It focuses on understanding the functions of various organ systems, tissues, and cells within the body, as well as how they interact with each other to maintain overall health and function.

Human physiology explores topics such as how we breathe, digest food, circulate blood, regulate temperature, and respond to stimuli. It provides insights into the complex mechanisms and processes that underlie bodily functions, both in health and disease.

Functions of The Major Organ Systems

- **The Cardiovascular System:**

  The cardiovascular system, also known as the circulatory system, is responsible for transporting blood, oxygen, nutrients, hormones, and waste products throughout the body. It consists of the heart, blood vessels (arteries, veins, and capillaries), and blood.

It's Key Functions Include:

→ The heart pumps blood to deliver oxygen and nutrients to various tissues and organs.

→ The arteries carry oxygen-rich blood away from the heart to the body's tissues.

→ The veins return oxygen-poor blood to the heart for oxygenation.

→ The capillaries facilitate the exchange of gases, nutrients, and waste products between blood and tissues.

- **Respiratory System:**

  The respiratory system is responsible for the exchange of gases, primarily oxygen and carbon dioxide, between the body and the environment. It includes the lungs and airways (trachea, bronchi, bronchioles), as well as muscles involved in breathing.

It's Key Functions Include:

→ The lungs inhale oxygen from the air and exhale carbon dioxide, thereby removing waste gases from the body.

→ The air passages facilitates gas exchanges by conducting air to and from the lungs.

→ Breathing muscles, such as the diaphragm and intercostal muscles, control the expansion and contraction of the lungs to enable inhalation and exhalation.

- **Nervous System:**

The nervous system controls and coordinates bodily activities and responses to internal and external stimuli. It includes the brain, spinal cord, nerves, and sensory organs (eyes, ears, skin).

It's Key Functions Include:

→ The brain processes sensory information, initiates voluntary movements, and regulates involuntary functions such as heart rate and digestion.

→ The spinal cord relays messages between the brain and peripheral nerves, facilitating sensory and motor functions.

→ Nerves in the body transmit electrical impulses to and from the various parts of the body, allowing for communication between cells, tissues, and organs.

- **Digestive System:**

  The digestive system is responsible for breaking down food into smaller molecules that can be absorbed and utilized by the body. It includes the mouth, esophagus, stomach, intestines, liver, pancreas, and gallbladder.

It's Key Functions Include:

→ The mouth and salivary glands begin the process of digestion by breaking down food into smaller pieces and mixing it with saliva.

→ The stomach secretes gastric juices that further break down food into a semi-liquid form called chyme.

→ The small intestine absorbs nutrients from digested food, while the large intestine absorbs water and electrolytes and forms feces for elimination.

- **Endocrine System:**

  The endocrine system regulates bodily functions and maintains homeostasis by secreting hormones into the bloodstream. It includes glands such as the pituitary, thyroid, adrenal, pancreas, and reproductive glands.

It's Key Functions Include:

→ Hormones act as chemical messengers that regulate metabolism, growth, development, reproduction, and stress response.

→ The pituitary gland controls other endocrine glands and secretes hormones that influence growth, development, and fluid balance.

→ The thyroid gland regulates metabolism and energy production, while the adrenal glands produce hormones involved in stress response and salt balance.

These major organ systems work together seamlessly to support the human body's functions, maintain homeostasis, and ensure overall health and well-being. Most importantly, the knowledge of their roles and interactions is essential for healthcare professionals to diagnose, treat, and prevent diseases and disorders.

How These Organs Work Together to Maintain Homeostasis and Support Overall Health

The physiology of humans is a complex system made up of numerous organs and organ systems, each with specific functions. While each system performs distinct roles, they also work together in a coordinated manner to maintain homeostasis and support overall health.

Homeostasis refers to the body's ability to maintain internal stability and balance despite external changes. Here's an in-depth exploration of how different organ systems collaborate to achieve homeostasis and promote overall health.

- **Integration of Organ Systems:**

The body's various organ systems are interconnected and interdependent, with each system influencing and being influenced by others. For example, the cardiovascular system transports oxygen and nutrients to tissues and removes metabolic waste products, supporting the metabolic activities of cells in the respiratory, digestive, and muscular systems.

- **Regulation of Internal Environment:**

  The organ systems work together to regulate the body's internal environment, including temperature, pH, fluid balance, and nutrient levels. For instance, the endocrine system secretes hormones that regulate blood glucose levels, while the kidneys maintain electrolyte balance and fluid volume through filtration and excretion.

- **Feedback Mechanisms:**

  Homeostasis is maintained through feedback mechanisms, which involve sensing changes in the internal environment and initiating responses to restore balance. Negative feedback loops are commonly employed where deviations from set points trigger corrective actions to return physiological parameters to normal levels.
  For example, if blood glucose levels rise after a meal, insulin is released by the pancreas to facilitate glucose uptake by cells, thereby lowering blood glucose levels back to the set point.

- **Coordination of Physiological Processes:**

  Organ systems coordinate their activities to meet the body's physiological demands and respond to internal and external stimuli. For instance, during exercise, the respiratory and cardiovascular systems collaborate to increase oxygen delivery to muscles and remove carbon dioxide, while the endocrine system releases hormones like adrenaline to enhance metabolism and energy production.

- **Adaptation to Environmental Changes:**

The body adapts to environmental changes through physiological responses mediated by various organ systems. For example, in response to exposure to high temperatures, the integumentary system releases sweat to dissipate heat, while blood vessels dilate to facilitate heat loss, maintaining body temperature within a narrow range.

- **Maintaining Cellular Function:**
  Homeostasis ensures that cells receive adequate oxygen, nutrients, and metabolic substrates while removing waste products to support cellular function and survival. The cardiovascular system transports oxygen and nutrients to tissues via the bloodstream, while the respiratory system facilitates gas exchange to supply oxygen and remove carbon dioxide.

Physiological Processes: Metabolism, Energy Production, and Waste Elimination

Physiological processes such as metabolism, energy production, and waste elimination are fundamental to maintaining the body's functions and overall health. Let's delve into each of these processes to see how they function.

- **Metabolism:**
Metabolism refers to the biochemical processes involved in converting food into energy and building blocks for cellular growth and repair. It consists of two main categories: catabolism, which breaks down molecules to release energy, and anabolism, which uses energy to build complex molecules.

Catabolic reactions involve the breakdown of complex molecules such as carbohydrates, fats, and proteins into simpler compounds, releasing energy in the process. For example, during cellular respiration, glucose is oxidized to produce ATP, the primary energy currency of cells.

While, anabolic reactions use energy to build complex molecules from simpler precursors, facilitating cellular growth, repair, and synthesis of biomolecules. Examples include protein synthesis, DNA replication, and glycogen formation.

It's metabolic pathways are tightly regulated to maintain homeostasis and meet the body's energy demands. Hormones, enzymes, and cellular signaling pathways play crucial roles in coordinating metabolic processes and responding to internal and external cues.

- **Energy Production:**

Energy production is the process by which cells generate ATP from glucose and oxygen. ATP is the energy currency used to power cellular activities. It consists of three main stages: glycolysis, the citric acid cycle, and oxidative phosphorylation.

Glycolysis occurs in the cytoplasm and involves the breakdown of glucose into pyruvate, producing a small amount of ATP and NADH. Pyruvate is then transported into the mitochondria for further oxidation.

The citric acid cycle takes place in the mitochondrial matrix and involves the oxidation of acetyl-CoA derived from pyruvate and fatty acids. It generates NADH and FADH2, which carries electrons to the electron transport chain.

While the oxidative phosphorylation occurs in the inner mitochondrial membrane and involves the transfer of electrons along the electron transport chain, coupled with the production of ATP via ATP synthase.

The oxygen serves as the final electron acceptor which forms water in the process. In addition to cellular respiration, energy can also be generated through other pathways such as anaerobic glycolysis (in the absence of oxygen) and fatty acid oxidation (beta-oxidation).

- **Waste Elimination:**

Waste elimination is the process by which the body removes metabolic by-products, toxins, and other unwanted substances to maintain internal homeostasis. It involves multiple organ systems, primarily the urinary, respiratory, digestive, and integumentary systems.

The urinary system eliminates metabolic wastes such as urea, creatinine, and uric acid from the blood through the production of urine by the kidneys. Urine is then excreted from the body via the ureters, bladder, and urethra.

The respiratory system removes carbon dioxide, a by-product of cellular respiration, from the blood through gas exchange in the lungs. The oxygen is taken up from the air and transported to cells for energy production, while carbon dioxide is expelled during exhalation.

The digestive system eliminates undigested food residues, metabolic wastes, and toxins through defecation. The liver detoxifies harmful substances and excretes waste products such as bile pigments into the bile, which is then eliminated via the feces.

The integumentary system, primarily the skin, eliminates metabolic wastes such as water, salts, and small amounts of urea through sweating. The sweat glands secrete sweat onto the skin's surface, where it evaporates and helps to regulate body temperature and remove wastes.

➤ Respiratory Physiology

Respiratory physiology is a field of study within physiology that focuses on how the respiratory system works. This includes understanding how our lungs, airways, and other respiratory organs function to breathe in oxygen and exhale carbon dioxide.

As a TEAS 7 exam candidate, grasping respiratory physiology is crucial as it often appears in the Science section, particularly in questions about human anatomy and physiology.

Most importantly, in the healthcare world, a solid understanding of respiratory physiology is vital for healthcare professionals like pulmonologists, anesthesiologists, and respiratory therapists because they rely on this knowledge to diagnose and treat respiratory conditions such as asthma, COPD, and pneumonia. Here is a simple rundown of Respiratory Physiology.

Functions of the Respiratory System: Gas Exchange, Ventilation, and Pulmonary Circulation

The respiratory system performs several essential functions that are crucial for sustaining life and maintaining homeostasis in the body. These functions include gas exchange, ventilation, and pulmonary circulation.

- **Gas Exchange:**

Gas exchange is the process by which oxygen is taken in from the air and carbon dioxide is expelled from the body. The primary function of the respiratory system is to facilitate the exchange of gases between the body and the environment.

This process involves the uptake of oxygen (O_2) from inhaled air and the elimination of carbon dioxide (CO_2) from the body.

In the lungs, oxygen from inhaled air diffuses from the alveoli (tiny air sacs) into the bloodstream, where it binds to hemoglobin in red blood cells for transport to cells throughout the body.

At the same time, the carbon dioxide produced by cellular metabolism also diffuses from the bloodstream into the alveoli to be exhaled.

- **Ventilation:**

Ventilation, or breathing, involves the movement of air into and out of the lungs. During inhalation (inspiration), the diaphragm and intercostal muscles contract, causing the chest cavity to expand.

This expansion lowers the air pressure in the lungs, allowing air to rush in from the atmosphere. While Exhalation (expiration) occurs when the diaphragm and intercostal muscles relax.

This causes the chest cavity to decrease in size and increases the air pressure in the lungs, for air to be expelled from the lungs.

- **Pulmonary Circulation:**

Pulmonary circulation is the circulation of blood between the heart and the lungs. This circulation is responsible for oxygenating blood and removing carbon dioxide, through the deoxygenated blood pumped from the right side of the heart into the lungs via the pulmonary arteries.

Right in the lungs, the blood vessels called pulmonary capillaries picks up oxygen and releases carbon dioxide through gas exchange in the alveoli. Then the oxygen diffuses into the bloodstream, while carbon dioxide diffuses out of the bloodstream into the alveoli.

The oxygenated blood returns to the heart via the pulmonary veins which is then pumped to the rest of the body to supply oxygen to tissues and organs.

These functions ensure that the body receives an adequate supply of oxygen for cellular respiration and removes waste carbon dioxide to maintain proper physiological balance.

Essential Mechanisms of Respiratory Physiology.

These are mechanisms essential for the physiological processes that govern breathing and the transport of oxygen and carbon dioxide in the body:

- **Breathing Control:**

This the process by which the respiratory center in the brainstem monitors and regulates breathing rate and depth in response to changes in oxygen, carbon dioxide, and pH levels in the blood.

The brainstem is specifically located in the medulla oblongata and pons. The primary drive to breathe is triggered by increased levels of carbon dioxide (hypercapnia) and decreased levels of oxygen (hypoxia) in the blood.

Chemoreceptors in the arteries and brainstem also sense these changes and send signals to the respiratory center to increase the rate and depth of breathing.

Additionally, other factors such as emotional state, physical activity, and temperature can influence breathing rate and rhythm through input from higher brain centers.

- **Oxygen Transport:**

This is the process by which oxygen is carried from the lungs to tissues throughout the body via the bloodstream, primarily bound to hemoglobin in red blood cells, to support cellular respiration and energy production.

Oxygen diffuses from the alveoli into the pulmonary capillaries, where it binds to hemoglobin molecules in red blood cells to form oxyhemoglobin.

Then, Oxyhemoglobin is carried by the circulatory system to tissues and organs, where oxygen is released from hemoglobin and diffuses into cells for cellular respiration. This is the process by which cells produce energy.

Also, carbon dioxide, the waste product of cellular metabolism is transported in the bloodstream primarily as bicarbonate ions (HCO_3-) dissolved in plasma. It is also bound to the hemoglobin and in the form of dissolved gas.

- **Carbon Dioxide Elimination:**

The process by which carbon dioxide, a waste product of cellular metabolism is removed from the body during respiration is through exhalation.

Carbon dioxide is transported in the bloodstream primarily as bicarbonate ions and is eliminated from the body to maintain acid-base balance and pH homeostasis.

A small portion of carbon dioxide is also converted to bicarbonate ions (HCO_3-) in red blood cells through the enzyme carbonic anhydrase. The bicarbonate ions are transported in the bloodstream to the lungs, where they are converted back to carbon dioxide and water, which is then exhaled.

It is worthy to note that the regulation of carbon dioxide levels in the blood is critical for maintaining acid-base balance and pH homeostasis.

This is because the excessive accumulation of carbon dioxide (hypercapnia) can lead to respiratory acidosis, while decreased levels of carbon dioxide (hypocapnia) can result in respiratory alkalosis.

Three Most Common Respiratory Disorders: Asthma, COPD, Respiratory Infections and Therapeutic Approaches For Managing These Conditions

Respiratory disorders encompass a wide range of conditions that affect the lungs, airways, and other components of the respiratory system, each with unique characteristics and management approaches.

Now, we'll talk about the three most common respiratory disorders: asthma, chronic obstructive pulmonary disease (COPD), and respiratory infections such as pneumonia and bronchitis.

Understanding these disorders and their management is crucial for healthcare professionals and students' preparing for the TEAS 7 exam because of the significant challenges it presents to the patients.

- **Asthma:**

Asthma is a chronic inflammatory condition characterized by reversible airflow obstruction and bronchospasm. Common symptoms include wheezing, shortness of breath, chest tightness, and coughing,

Asthma symptoms can be triggered by factors like allergens (e.g., pollen, pet dander), respiratory infections, exercise, cold air, smoke, and air pollutants.

This could lead to acute respiratory distress and require prompt intervention. Asthma treatment typically involves a combination of long-term control medications (e.g., inhaled corticosteroids, bronchodilators) to prevent symptoms and quick rescue medications (e.g., short-acting bronchodilators) for acute relief during exacerbations.

It is also important for healthcare officials to educate the patients on asthma triggers, as well as proper inhaler techniques. This is to effectively manage the asthmatic condition.

- **Chronic Obstructive Pulmonary Disease (COPD):**

COPD is a progressive lung disease characterized by airflow limitation and irreversible damage to lung tissue. It is typically caused by long-term exposure to irritants such as cigarette smoke.

It's symptoms manifest as chronic cough, excessive sputum production, dyspnea (shortness of breath), and reduced exercise tolerance.

There are two main types of COPD condition: Chronic bronchitis, involving inflammation and mucus production in the airways, and Emphysema, which involves damage to the lung tissue and alveoli.

This condition can be managed through therapeutic treatments that aim to relieve the symptoms, improve quality of life, and prevent futher exacerbations.

They includes smoking cessation (Quitting smoking), pulmonary rehabilitation, bronchodilator medications (e.g., long-acting beta-agonists, anticholinergics), corticosteroids, oxygen therapy, and vaccination against respiratory infections.

- **Respiratory Infections:**

Respiratory infections such as pneumonia (inflammation of the lungs), bronchitis (inflammation of the bronchial tubes), and influenza(the flu), are caused by bacteria, viruses, fungi, or other pathogens.

They affect different parts of the respiratory tract, leading to symptoms like cough, fever, chest pain, and difficulty breathing.

These respiratory infections treatment depends on the pathogen involved and may include antibiotics for bacterial infections, antiviral medications for influenza, and supportive care measures such as rest, hydration, and fever management. It's preventive measures include: vaccination, hand hygiene, and avoiding close contact with individuals who are sick.

➢ Chemistry

Chemistry is the branch of science that studies the properties, composition, and interactions of matter, which is anything that has mass and occupies space.

It explores the structure of atoms and molecules, the changes they undergo, and the energy involved in these transformations. Chemistry is all around us, influencing everything from the air we breathe to the food we eat and the materials we use in our daily lives and environment.

Chemistry is so important that it cannot be switched for anything else. Here are a few key reasons why it matters.

Importance of Chemistry

- **Understanding Matter:** Chemistry helps us understand the nature of different substances, their properties, and how they behave with each other. This knowledge is essential for designing new materials, developing medicines, preparing meals, and solving real-world problems.

- **Advancing Technology**: Chemistry plays a crucial role in the development of new materials, medicines, and technologies that improve our quality of life. It contributes to innovations in fields such as healthcare, energy production, materials science, electronics, agriculture, and manufacturing. From new drug formulations to cleaner energy sources, chemistry plays a critical role in improving our lives.

- **Environmental Protection:** Chemistry provides insights into environmental issues such as pollution, climate change, and resource conservation. It helps us understand the impact of human activities on the environment, and by understanding chemical processes in the environment, we can develop strategies to mitigate harmful effects and promote sustainability.

- **Health and Medicine:** Chemistry is fundamental to pharmaceuticals and healthcare as a whole. It allows us to develop drugs to treat diseases, understand biochemical processes in the body, and diagnose medical conditions through techniques like blood tests and imaging.

- **Food and Nutrition:** Chemistry informs our understanding of nutrition and food safety, including the composition of nutrients, food additives, and contaminants, as well as the processes involved in food preservation and cooking.

- **Energy Production:** Chemistry is central to energy production technologies, including fossil fuels, nuclear energy, and renewable sources such as solar and wind power. By studying chemical reactions and energy conversion processes, we can develop more efficient and sustainable energy solutions.

- **Diagnostic Techniques:** Chemistry contributes to diagnostic techniques used in healthcare. From simple chemical tests to advanced imaging technologies, chemistry enables the detection and monitoring of diseases, assessment of physiological functions, and evaluation of treatment efficacy. Diagnostic tests rely on chemical reactions and principles to detect biomarkers, pathogens, and other indicators of health or disease.

Overall, chemistry is a fundamental part of science that touches virtually every aspect of our lives, as it contributes to advancements in technology, healthcare, agriculture, and environmental protection. It also provides the foundation for addressing global challenges and improving the well-being of society.

In the context of the TEAS 7 exam, chemistry is a significant component of the Science section. Students are tested on their understanding of basic chemistry concepts such as atomic structure, chemical bonding, reactions, and the periodic table.

Also, they may encounter questions that apply chemistry principles to healthcare scenarios that requires them to apply their knowledge to solve problems and analyze information effectively.

So, by mastering chemistry concepts, TEAS 7 students can excel in the exam and acquire valuable knowledge applicable to their future careers in healthcare. Whether pursuing roles as nurses, medical laboratory technicians, or other healthcare professionals, a strong foundation in chemistry equips students with the essential skills to understand the chemical basis of biological processes, pharmacology, and medical technology.

➤ Atomic Structure and The Periodic Table

Atomic structure refers to the composition and arrangement of particles within an atom. They are the smallest units of matter that retain the properties of an element. Atoms, the basic building blocks of matter, consist of three main subatomic particles: protons, neutrons, and electrons.

Protons and neutrons are found in the nucleus, located at the center of the atom, while electrons orbit the nucleus in distinct energy levels called electron shells. Protons are positively charged particles found in the nucleus of an atom.

The number of protons in the nucleus determines the atomic number of an atom, and it identifies the element's identity and its unique properties. It is referred to as the atomic number (Z).

Neutrons are neutral particles found in the nucleus alongside protons. They contribute to the atom's mass but do not affect its chemical behavior or properties. While, Electrons are negatively charged particles that orbit the nucleus in specific energy levels or electron shells.

The outermost shell, known as the valence shell, determines the atom's chemical behavior. They are also responsible for chemical bonding and interactions between atoms.

The arrangement of electrons in the electron shells follows certain rules, including the Aufbau principle, Pauli exclusion principle, and Hund's rule. These rules dictate the filling order of electrons in orbitals within the electron shells.

➤ The Periodic Table

The periodic table is a tabular arrangement that provides valuable information of chemical elements, organized by their atomic number, atomic symbol, electron configuration, and recurring chemical properties.

It consists of rows called periods and columns known as groups or families. The more you move across a period from left to right, the atomic number increases, and the chemical properties change gradually.

Also, elements within the same group share similar chemical behaviors and properties due to their comparable electron configurations. The periodic table allow scientists predict the behavior of elements and their compounds, facilitating research, experimentation, and practical applications in fields like chemistry, physics, and materials science.

➤ Its Key Concepts and Trends

When you understand the atomic structure and the periodic table, you'll be able to identify key concepts and trends like:

- **Atomic Number:** The number of protons in the nucleus determines the atomic number, which uniquely identifies each element.
- **Atomic Mass:** The sum of protons and neutrons in the nucleus gives the atomic mass, which is typically expressed in atomic mass units (amu).
- **Electron Configuration:** The arrangement of electrons in the electron shells determines an element's chemical properties and reactivity.
- **Periodic Trends:** Trends such as atomic radius, ionization energy, electron affinity, and electronegativity can be observed across periods and groups in the periodic table. These trends provide valuable insights into element behavior and chemical bonding.

Overall, the atomic structure and the periodic table serve as the foundation for understanding the behavior and properties of elements and their interactions in chemical reactions. They are essential tools for chemists, educators, and students. Most importantly, it guides research, discovery, and innovation in the field of chemistry.

Chemical Bonding: Covalent, Ionic, and Hydrogen Bonds (How Atoms Combine to Form Molecules Through Different Types of Bonds)

➤ Chemical Bonding

Chemical bonding is a fundamental concept in chemistry that governs the formation of molecules and compounds. It refers to the attractive forces that hold atoms together in molecules or compounds.

These bonds are formed either by the sharing or transfer of electrons between atoms, leading to the formation of stable structures. The three main types of chemical bonds include:

- **Ionic Bonds:** Ionic bonds form when one or more electrons are transferred from one atom to another, resulting in the formation of positively and negatively charged ions. These ions are held together by the strong electrostatic attraction between opposite charges.

  For example, sodium (Na) and chlorine (Cl) atoms can form an ionic bond to create sodium chloride (NaCl), commonly known as table salt. Ionic bonds typically occur between atoms with significantly different electronegativities, where one atom has a strong tendency to lose electrons (cation) and the other has a strong tendency to gain electrons (anion). The bonds are relatively strong and often form crystalline structures in solid-state compounds.

  Furthermore, the transfer of electrons results in the formation of ions with complete outer electron shells, making them more stable than the original atoms. These ions arrange themselves in a repeating pattern to form an ionic lattice.

- **Covalent Bonds:** Covalent bonds occur when atoms share electrons to achieve a stable electron configuration. This sharing allows atoms to complete their outer electron shells, typically composed of eight electrons (the octet rule), resulting in a more stable arrangement.

  Unlike ionic bonds, where electrons are transferred, covalent bonds involve the mutual attraction of nuclei for shared electrons. Covalent bonds are typically stronger than ionic bonds and can be either polar or nonpolar, depending on the electronegativity difference between the atoms involved.

  For instance, in a water molecule (H_2O), oxygen shares electrons with two hydrogen atoms through covalent bonds.

  Covalent bonds can be classified into two types: polar and nonpolar. In polar covalent bonds, electrons are shared unequally between atoms due to differences in electronegativity, which results in a partial positive or negative charge on each atom.

While, nonpolar covalent bonds involve the equal sharing of electrons between atoms. This results in no net charge on the atoms. This type of bonds are prevalent in organic compounds and play a crucial role in the structure and function of biomolecules such as proteins, carbohydrates, and lipids.

Examples of molecules held together by covalent bonds include water (H_2O), carbon dioxide (CO_2), and methane (CH_4).

- **Hydrogen Bonds:** Hydrogen bonds are a type of weak intermolecular force that occurs when a hydrogen atom with a partial positive charge is attracted to an electronegative atom with a partial negative charge.

  Although hydrogen bonds are weaker than covalent or ionic bonds, they play a crucial role in the structure and properties of many molecules, particularly those containing hydrogen, oxygen, nitrogen, or fluorine.

  This type of bonds contribute to the unique properties of water, such as its high boiling point, surface tension, and ability to dissolve a wide range of substances.

  Additionally, hydrogen bonds are important in biological molecules such as proteins and nucleic acids, where they help stabilize the three-dimensional structure and facilitate specific molecular interactions.

These three main types of chemical bonds and how they form is essential for explaining the structure, properties, and behavior of molecules in various chemical and biological systems. In the healthcare world, this knowledge is essential for understanding drug interactions, biochemical processes, and the molecular basis of diseases.

➢ **Chemical Reactions**

Chemical reactions are processes where substances go through chemical changes that result in the formation of new substances with different chemical properties.

In a chemical reaction, one or more reactants interact to form one or more products. In these reactions, atoms are rearranged, and chemical bonds are broken and formed. This rearrangement leads to the creation of new combinations of elements, resulting in the formation of products from reactants.

Chemical reactions can be represented using chemical equations, which show the reactants on the left side and the products on the right side. They are separated by an arrow indicating the direction of the reaction.

The coefficients in front of the chemical formulas indicate the relative amounts of each substance involved in the reaction, while the subscripts within the formulas represent the number of atoms of each element in the compound.

Chemical reactions can be classified into various types based on the nature of the reactants and products, as well as the rearrangement of atoms during the reaction. Some common types of chemical reactions include:

- **Synthesis Reactions:** Also known as combination reactions, synthesis reactions involve the combination of two or more reactants to form a single product. In these reactions, two or more substances combine to form a more complex product.

  The general form of a synthesis reaction is A + B → AB, where A and B are reactants and AB is the product.

  For example, the reaction of hydrogen gas (H_2) with oxygen gas (O_2) to form water (H_2O) is a synthesis reaction: $2H_2 + O_2 \rightarrow 2H_2O$.

  Synthesis reactions are common in nature and play a significant role in the formation of various compounds and molecules.

- **Decomposition Reactions:** Decomposition reactions involve the breakdown of a single reactant or compound into two or more products or simpler substances. In these reactions, a single reactant decomposes to form multiple products. The general form of a decomposition reaction is $AB \rightarrow A + B$, where AB is the reactant and A and B are the products.

  An example of a decomposition reaction is the breakdown of hydrogen peroxide (H_2O_2) into water (H_2O) and oxygen gas (O_2): $2H_2O_2 \rightarrow 2H_2O + O_2$. This kind of reactions are important for processes such as digestion, decomposition of organic matter, and the breakdown of pollutants in the environment.

- **Single Replacement Reactions:** In single replacement reactions, one element replaces another element in a compound which results in the formation of a new compound and a different element.

  The general form of a single replacement reaction is $A + BC \rightarrow AC + B$, where A is the replacing element, BC is the compound, AC is the new compound, and B is the other element.

  For instance, the reaction of zinc metal (Zn) with hydrochloric acid (HCl) to produce zinc chloride ($ZnCl_2$) and hydrogen gas (H_2): $Zn + 2HCl \rightarrow ZnCl_2 + H_2$.

- **Double Replacement Reactions:** Double replacement reactions involve the exchange of ions between two compounds that results in the formation of two new compounds.

  The general form of a double replacement reaction is $AB + CD \rightarrow AD + CB$, where AB and CD are the reactants, and AD and CB are the products. A good example is the reaction between sodium chloride (NaCl) and silver nitrate ($AgNO_3$) to form sodium nitrate ($NaNO_3$) and silver chloride (AgCl): $NaCl + AgNO_3 \rightarrow NaNO_3 + AgCl$.

- **Combustion Reactions:** Combustion reactions involve the rapid reaction of a substance with oxygen gas (O2) to produce heat and light. An example is the combustion of methane (CH4) in the presence of oxygen to form carbon dioxide (CO2) and water (H2O): $CH_4 + 2O_2 \rightarrow CO_2 + 2H_2O$.

- **Acid-Base Reactions:** Acid-base reactions, also known as neutralization reactions, occur when an acid reacts with a base to form a salt and water. These reactions involve the transfer of protons (H+ ions) between the acid and base.

  An example of an acid-base reaction is the reaction between hydrochloric acid (HCl) and sodium hydroxide (NaOH) to form sodium chloride (NaCl) and water (H2O): $HCl + NaOH \rightarrow NaCl + H_2O$.

  Acid-base reactions are important for the maintanance of pH balance in biological systems and are commonly used in various industrial processes.

- **Oxidation-Reduction (Redox) Reactions:** Oxidation-reduction reactions, or redox reactions, involve the transfer of electrons between reactants. In these reactions, one substance undergoes oxidation (loses electrons) while another undergoes reduction (gains electrons).

  An example of a redox reaction is the combustion of methane (CH4) in the presence of oxygen (O2) to form carbon dioxide (CO2) and water (H2O): $CH_4 + 2O_2 \rightarrow CO_2 + 2H_2O$.

  Redox reactions play a critical role in energy production, metabolism, corrosion, and many other chemical processes.

Properties of Matter: Characteristics of Different States of Matter (Solids, Liquids, Gases, and Solutions)

➢ Properties of Matter

Properties of matter are like the unique traits that help us understand what things are made of and how they behave. They are the characteristics or attributes that describe the physical and chemical behavior of substances.

These properties can be observed or measured and they help classify and identify different types of matter. Some common properties of matter include:

- **Physical Properties:**

Physical properties describe the characteristics of matter that can be observed or measured without changing the substance's chemical composition. Examples include:

→ **Mass:** Mass is like how heavy something is. It is the amount of matter in an object and it is usually measured in grams or kilograms. For example, it tells us how many pills are in a medicine bottle or how much food is on a plate.

→ **Volume:** Volume helps us figure out how big or small things are. It is the amount of space occupied by an object or substance and it is typically measured in liters or cubic meters. For example, think of it like filling up a glass of water – the amount of water you pour in shows its volume.

→ **Density:** Density is a bit tricky. It's about how tightly packed the particles in a substance are. For instance, a heavy metal block. However, something less dense has fewer particles in the same space, like a balloon filled with air. Density is the mass of a substance per unit volume.

→ **Color:** Color is the visual appearance of a substance when it interacts with light.

→ **Texture:** This is the feel or appearance of the surface of a substance. It could be smooth, rough, or powdery.

→ **Melting Point:** This is the temperature at which a solid substance changes into a liquid.

→ **Boiling Point:** This is the temperature at which a liquid substance changes into a gas.
→ **State of Matter:** This is whether a substance exists as a solid, liquid, or gas under specific conditions of temperature and pressure. Let's dive deeper into the different states if matter.

- **Solids:**

Solids have a definite shape and volume. The particles in a solid are tightly packed together and vibrate in place. They have strong attractive forces between them, giving them in a rigid structure. Solids don't move around freely like in liquids or gases.

Characteristics:
→ **Shape:** Solids have a fixed shape, meaning they maintain their form regardless of the container they're in.
→ **Volume:** They also have a fixed volume, meaning they don't change their amount of space they take up.
→ **Density:** Solids are typically denser than liquids and gases because their particles are closely packed together.
→ **Rigidity:** Solids are rigid and resist changes in shape and volume. Examples: Examples of solids include rocks, metals, wood, and ice.

- **Liquids:**

Liquids have a definite volume but take the shape of their container. The particles in a liquid are close together but can move past each other, this allows the liquid to flow.

Characteristics:
→ **Shape:** Liquids take the shape of the container they're in, but they maintain a constant volume.
→ **Volume:** Liquids have a fixed volume, meaning they don't change their amount of space they take up.
→ **Fluidity:** Liquids flow and can be poured, making them fluids.

→ **Surface Tension:** Liquids have surface tension, which causes them to form droplets and allows them to bead up on surfaces. Examples of liquids include water, milk, oil, and alcohol.

- **Gases:**

Gases have neither a definite shape nor volume. The particles in a gas are far apart and move freely in all directions, colliding with each other and the walls of their container.

Characteristics:

→ **Shape:** Gases take the shape of the container they're in and expand to fill the entire volume of the container.

→ **Volume:** Gases do not have a fixed volume and can expand or contract to fit the size of their container.

→ **Compressibility:** Gases are highly compressible, meaning %™© volume can be reduced under pressure.

→ **Diffusion:** Gases mix and spread out evenly when not confined, a process known as diffusion. Examples of gases include oxygen, nitrogen, carbon dioxide, and helium.

- **Solutions:**

Solutions are homogeneous mixtures composed of two or more substances, where one substance is dissolved in another substance. The substance present in the largest amount is called the solvent, while the dissolved substance is called the solute.

Characteristics:

→ **Homogeneity:** Solutions are uniform throughout, meaning they have the same composition and properties at all points.

→ **Dissolvability:** Solutes dissolve in solvents to form solutions, and the resulting mixture is typically transparent or translucent.

→ **Concentration:** The concentration of a solution refers to the amount of solute dissolved in the solvent, usually expressed as a percentage or molarity. Examples of solutions include saltwater (sodium chloride dissolved in water), sugar water (sucrose dissolved in water), and vinegar (acetic acid dissolved in water).

➤ Chemical Properties

Chemical properties describe how a substance interacts with other substances or undergoes chemical changes to form new substances. Examples include:

- **Flammability:** This is the ability of a substance to burn or combust when exposed to heat or flame. Some things, like wood or paper, are very flammable, while others, like metal or glass, hardly ever catch fire.
- **Reactivity:** This is how readily a substance reacts with other substances to form new compounds. For example, when you mix vinegar (an acid) with baking soda, it fizzes up because of a chemical reaction.
- **Acidity/Basicity:** This tells us if something is acidic (like lemon juice) or basic (like soap). It is the ability of a substance to react with acids or bases and form salts.
- **Toxicity:** Toxicity is all about how harmful something can be to living things. It is the negative effects of a substance on living organisms when ingested, inhaled, or absorbed. Substances like bleach or pesticides can be toxic if not handled carefully.
- **Corrosiveness:** The ability of a substance to deteriorate or degrade other materials through chemical reactions.

Organic & Biochemistry: The Chemistry of Living Organisms, Structure and Function of Biological Molecules (Carbohydrates, Lipids, Proteins, and Nucleic Acids)

Organic and biochemistry deals with the study of carbon-containing compounds and their roles in living organisms. Let's talk about some basic principles relevant to living organisms:

➤ Carbon Chemistry

Carbon atoms possess unique properties that enable them to form stable covalent bonds with other atoms, including carbon itself and other elements such as hydrogen, oxygen, nitrogen, and sulfur.

This versatility allows carbon to serve as the backbone for a vast array of organic molecules with complex structures and functions. Organic molecules often exhibit structural isomerism, where compounds with the same molecular formula have different arrangements of atoms, leading to diverse chemical properties and biological functions.

• Functional Groups:

Functional groups are specific arrangements of atoms within organic molecules that impart distinct chemical properties and reactivity to the molecule. Each functional group has characteristic chemical properties and can participate in specific types of chemical reactions.

For example, the hydroxyl group (-OH) imparts hydrophilic properties to molecules and can participate in hydrogen bonding, while the carbonyl group (>C=O) is involved in reactions such as oxidation and reduction. Other examples of functional groups include hydroxyl (-OH), carbonyl (C=O), amino (-NH2), and carboxyl (-COOH

• Macromolecules:

Organic molecules can be classified into four main categories: carbohydrates, lipids, proteins, and nucleic acids. Here is a detailed explanation on these molecules:

→ **Carbohydrates:** Carbohydrates are composed of carbon, hydrogen, and oxygen atoms. They have a basic structure of carbon atoms arranged in a chain, with hydrogen and hydroxyl (OH) groups attached. Carbohydrates serve as the primary source of energy for cells, particularly glucose. They also play roles in cell structure and cell recognition.

→ **Lipids:** Lipids are diverse molecules, including fats, oils, and phospholipids. They are composed mainly of carbon and hydrogen atoms, with some oxygen atoms. Lipids serve as energy storage molecules, insulate and protect organs, and form the structure of cell membranes. Additionally, certain lipids act as signaling molecules and are involved in hormone production.

→ **Proteins:** Proteins are made up of long chains of amino acids linked together by peptide bonds. Each amino acid has a unique side chain that determines its properties.

Proteins have diverse functions in the body, including enzyme catalysis, structural support, transport of molecules, immune response, and cell signaling.

Examples include enzymes that facilitate chemical reactions, antibodies that defend against pathogens, and collagen that provides structural support to tissues.

Nucleic Acids: Nucleic acids, such as DNA and RNA, are composed of nucleotide units. Each nucleotide consists of a phosphate group, a sugar molecule (deoxyribose or ribose), and a nitrogenous base (adenine, guanine, cytosine, or thymine/uracil).

Nucleic acids store and transmit genetic information. DNA carries the genetic instructions for protein synthesis and is inherited from parents to offspring. RNA plays roles in protein synthesis and gene regulation.

• **Metabolism:**

Metabolism refers to all the biochemical reactions that occur within an organism to maintain life. It consists of two main processes: catabolism, which breaks down complex molecules into simpler ones to release energy, and anabolism, which synthesizes complex molecules from simpler ones, requiring energy input. Metabolism is tightly regulated to maintain cellular homeostasis and respond to changing environmental conditions, ensuring that cells have the energy and resources they need to function properly.

- **Enzymes:**

Enzymes are biological catalysts that accelerate chemical reactions by lowering the activation energy required for the reaction to proceed. Enzymes are highly specific, often recognizing and binding to specific substrates to facilitate their conversion into products. Enzyme activity is influenced by factors such as temperature, pH, substrate concentration, and the presence of inhibitors or activators. They lay crucial roles in virtually all biochemical pathways, regulating the rate of reactions and ensuring metabolic efficiency.

- **Biochemical Pathways:**

Biochemical pathways are sequences of enzymatic reactions that occur sequentially within cells to convert substrates into products. They perform specific functions such as energy production, biosynthesis, and cellular signaling.

These biochemical pathways are also highly organized and tightly regulated to maintain metabolic balance and respond to physiological demands. Examples of biochemical pathways include glycolysis, the citric acid cycle, gluconeogenesis, and the pentose phosphate pathway.

When these pathways are studied, they provide insights into how cells extract energy from nutrients, synthesize essential molecules, and regulate cellular processes.

These fundamental concepts in organic and biochemistry gives a deeper understanding of the molecular basis of life processes and the mechanisms underlying cellular function, metabolism, and organismal physiology.

This knowledge is indispensable in fields such as medicine, pharmacology, bioengineering, and biotechnology, where it informs research, drug development, and clinical practice.

➤ Biology

Biology is the scientific study of living organisms and how they interact with each other and their environments. This science subject is made up of a wide range of topics, from the structure and function of cells to the behavior of entire ecosystems.

In essence, biology seeks to understand the fundamental principles that govern life processes and the diversity of life on Earth.

In the healthcare world, it serves as the foundation for understanding human anatomy, physiology, genetics, and disease. This is because healthcare professionals rely on biological principles to diagnose illnesses, develop treatments, and promote health and wellness.

For example, the knowledge of biology helps physicians understand how the body responds to pathogens and medications, while biologists study the genetic basis of diseases to develop targeted therapies.

For you a TEAS 7 student, biology is a key subject area tested on the examination and your questions may cover topics such as cellular biology, genetics, ecology, and human anatomy and physiology.

So, understanding these concepts is essential for success on the exam and for pursuing your career in any healthcare-related field of your choice. Now, as you continue reading, you'll see a comprehensive yet concise explaination of these concepts with examples for easy understanding.

Cell Biology: The Structure and Function of Cells

Cell biology, also known as cytology, is the branch of biology that focuses on the study of cells. It studies the smallest units of life—cells, which are the basic structural and functional units of all living organisms.

Cells are incredibly diverse, ranging from simple prokaryotic cells, like bacteria, to complex eukaryotic cells found in plants, animals, fungi, and protists.

Cell biology talks about how cells are structured, how they function, including the various organelles within cells, and how they interact with each other and their environment.

At the heart of cell biology is the exploration of cell structure. Cells are surrounded by a plasma membrane, a selectively permeable barrier that separates the cell from its external environment and they are highly organized structures containing numerous organelles, each with specific functions.

These organelles include the nucleus, which houses the cell's genetic material and information (DNA), which directs cellular activities and serves as the blueprint for protein synthesis.

Mitochondria, the powerhouses of the cell responsible for producing ATP - the cell's primary source of energy, produces it through aerobic cellular respiration and converts nutrients into usable energy molecules.

The **Endoplasmic reticulum** is involved in protein synthesis and lipid metabolism, while the Golgi apparatus, is responsible for processing and packaging proteins for transport to their final destinations (secretion).

Lysosomes function as the cell's recycling centers. It contain enzymes for breaking down waste materials, degrading and recycling cellular waste and damaged organelles.

Chloroplasts in plant cells perform photosynthesis, converting light energy into chemical energy in the form of glucose. Now let's go into all these in detail.

- **Structure of Cells**

- **Plasma Membrane (Cell Membrane):** The plasma membrane, or cell membrane, is a thin, flexible phospholipid bilayer (barrier) that surrounds the cell. It separates its internal contents from the external environment and it contains more of phospholipids, proteins, and carbohydrates.

  The phospholipid bilayer provides the membrane with its basic structure, with hydrophilic (water-attracting) heads facing outward and hydrophobic (water-repelling) tails facing inward.

  This regulates the passage of substances in and out of the cell, allowing nutrients to enter and waste products to exit while maintaining internal conditions.

- **Cytoplasm:** The cytoplasm is a gel-like substance that fills the cell interior and surrounds the organelles. It consists of water, salts, and organic molecules, providing a medium for cellular activities and supporting the organelles.

  It also contains various organelles, such as the endoplasmic reticulum, Golgi apparatus, mitochondria, and ribosomes, which carry out specific functions crucial for the cell's survival and function.

- **Nucleus:** The nucleus is a prominent organelle often referred to as the control center of the cell. It houses the cell's genetic material in the form of chromatin (chromosomes), which consists of DNA and associated proteins.

  It is also surrounded by a double membrane called the nuclear envelope, which contains pores that regulate the passage of materials between the nucleus and the cytoplasm. And within the nucleus is the nucleolus, where ribosomal RNA (rRNA) is synthesized and assembled with proteins to form ribosomes.

  The nucleus directs cellular activities by regulating gene expression and coordinating processes such as growth, metabolism, and reproduction.

- **Organelles:** Organelles are specialized structures within the cell that perform specific functions. Let talk more about them:

→ **Mitochondria:** Mitochondria are often called the powerhouses of the cell because they generate energy through cellular respiration, converting nutrients like glucose and oxygen into adenosine triphosphate (ATP), the cell's primary energy currency.

→ **Endoplasmic Reticulum (ER):** The endoplasmic reticulum is a network of membrane-bound tubes and sacs involved in protein and lipid synthesis with rough ER having ribosomes attached to its surface and smooth ER lacking ribosomes. It is also responsible for the transportation of molecules within the cell.

→ **Golgi Apparatus:** The Golgi apparatus modifies, sorts, and packages proteins and lipids into vesicles synthesized in the endoplasmic reticulum for secretion or delivery to other cellular locations.

→ **Lysosomes:** Lysosomes are membrane-bound vesicles containing digestive enzymes responsible for breaking down cellular waste, foreign substances, and damaged organelles.

→ **Chloroplasts (in plant cells):** Chloroplasts are unique to plant cells and are the site of photosynthesis, where light energy is converted into chemical energy in the form of glucose. That is, they use sunlight, water, and carbon dioxide to produce glucose and oxygen.

→ **Cytoskeleton:** The cytoskeleton is a network of protein filaments, including microtubules, microfilaments, and intermediate filaments, that provide structural support, maintain cell shape, and facilitate cell movement.

➤ **Functions of Cells**

The functions of cells include the following:

→ **Metabolism:** Cells carry out metabolic processes to maintain life, including energy production, biosynthesis of molecules (e.g., proteins, lipids), and the breakdown of nutrients for energy. These processes occur within specialized organelles and are regulated by enzymes.

→ **Homeostasis:** Cells maintain internal stability and balance, or homeostasis, by regulating their internal environment. This involves controlling factors such as pH, temperature, ion concentrations, and nutrient levels to ensure optimal conditions for cellular function and survival.

→ **Reproduction:** Cells reproduce through processes like cell division, which includes mitosis and meiosis. Cell division allows organisms to grow, repair damaged tissues, and produce offspring through asexual or sexual reproduction.

→ **Communication:** Cells communicate with each other through chemical signals, such as hormones, neurotransmitters, and signaling molecules. Cell-to-cell communication allows cells to coordinate their activities, respond to external stimuli, and regulate physiological processes.

→ **Differentiation:** During development, cells undergo differentiation, becoming specialized to perform specific functions within tissues and organs. This process involves changes in gene expression and cell morphology, leading to the formation of diverse cell types with distinct structures and functions.

→

➤ **Cellular Processes**

Cell biology also talks about cellular processes. Cellular processes are the numerous coordinated activities that occur within cells and allows them to carry out essential functions necessary for life.

These processes involve various organelles, molecules, and pathways working together to maintain cellular homeostasis, respond to stimuli, and carry out specialized functions.

Here are some key cellular processes that you should know as a TEAS 7 student:

- **Cellular Respiration:**

Cellular respiration is a complex biochemical process that occurs in eukaryotic cells, such as those in animals and plants. It is the process by which cells generate ATP (adenosine triphosphate), the primary energy currency of the cell, through the breakdown of glucose molecules.

Although in multiple stages, the process begins with glycolysis, which takes place in the cytoplasm and involves the breakdown of glucose into two molecules of pyruvate, producing a small amount of ATP and NADH.

The pyruvate then enters the mitochondria, where it undergoes further oxidation through the citric acid cycle (Krebs cycle) to generate more NADH and FADH2, along with ATP and carbon dioxide.

The electrons carried by NADH and FADH2 are then transferred to the electron transport chain, located in the inner mitochondrial membrane, where they drive the synthesis of ATP through oxidative phosphorylation.

Overall, cellular respiration produces a total of 36-38 ATP molecules per glucose molecule which provides the cell with the energy it needs to carry out various metabolic processes (cellular activities).

- **Photosynthesis:**

Photosynthesis is a vital process that occurs in chloroplasts, primarily in the thylakoid membranes and stroma, which is found in the cells of plants, algae, and some bacteria.

It is the process by which these plants, algae, and bacteria convert light energy into chemical energy in the form of glucose. The process begins with the absorption of light by chlorophyll molecules in the thylakoid membranes of chloroplasts, which triggers the light-dependent reactions.

Photosynthesis consists of two main stages: the light-dependent reactions, which capture light energy and convert it into chemical energy in the form of ATP and NADPH, and the **light-independent reactions** which use the ATP and NADPH to synthesize glucose from carbon dioxide.

During the light-dependent reactions, light energy is used to split water molecules into oxygen, protons, and electrons. Then the electrons are then transported through a series of protein complexes, generating ATP and NADPH.

The ATP and NADPH generated from the light-dependent reactions are used in the light-independent reactions, also known as the Calvin cycle, to fix carbon dioxide and synthesize glucose.

Overall, photosynthesis produces oxygen as a byproduct and converts carbon dioxide and water into glucose, providing energy for plant growth and oxygen for aerobic respiration.

- **Protein Synthesis:**

Protein synthesis is the process by which cells make proteins that are essential for various cellular functions, such as structural support, cell signaling, and enzymatic activity.

It occurs in two main stages: transcription and translation. The process begins with transcription, which occurs in the nucleus, where the DNA sequence of a gene is transcribed into a complementary RNA molecule called messenger RNA (mRNA).

The mRNA molecules then exit the nucleus and enter the cytoplasm, where translation takes place on ribosomes. During translation, the mRNA sequence is decoded by ribosomes, and amino acids are brought to the ribosome by transfer RNA (tRNA) molecules, which have anticodons complementary to the mRNA codons.

The amino acids are joined together in a specific sequence to form a polypeptide chain, which folds into a functional protein with a specific three-dimensional structure.

- **Cell Division:**

Cell division is the process by which cells reproduce and proliferate, allowing for growth, development, and repair of tissues. It involves the replication and distribution of genetic material to daughter cells.

Cell division occurs in two main stages: mitosis and cytokinesis. The process begins with interphase, during which the cell grows, replicates its DNA, and prepares for division.

Cell division then proceeds through mitosis, which involves the division of the nucleus, and cytokinesis, and of the cytoplasm. Mitosis is the division of the nucleus, resulting in two daughter nuclei that are genetically identical to the parent nucleus.

It is divided into several stages: prophase, metaphase, anaphase, and telophase, each characterized by specific changes in chromosome structure and organization. While cytokinesis is the division of the cytoplasm between the two daughter cells and it's results form two separate genetically identical daughter cells.

- **Cell Signaling:**

Cell signaling is the process by which cells communicate with each other to coordinate their activities and respond to extracellular stimuli. It involves the binding of signaling molecules, such as hormones or neurotransmitters to receptors on the cell surface or within the cell.

This initiates a series of intracellular signaling cascades. These signaling cascades involve the activation of various proteins, enzymes, and second messengers that relay the signal from the cell surface to the nucleus where they regulate gene expression and other cellular responses.

Cell signaling plays a crucial role in a wide range of physiological processes, including development, growth, metabolism, immune response, and cell differentiation.

Genetics: Inheritance Patterns, DNA Structure, and The Mechanisms of Gene Expression and Regulation

In genetics, there are fundamental concepts that would help you understand how traits are passed from one generation to the next and how genes function within organisms are inheritance patterns, DNA structure, and the mechanisms of gene expression and regulation.
Let's explain these starting with a comprehensive explanation of genetics.

Genetics is the branch of biology that focuses on the study of genes, heredity, and variation in living organisms. Genetics looks at how traits, like eye color or height, get passed from parents to kids.

It talks about the transmission of traits from one generation to the next, the molecular mechanisms underlying inheritance, and how genes influences and shapes an organism's characteristics.

Genes are segments of DNA that contain specific instructions for making proteins or functional RNA molecules. Genes are organized along chromosomes, a thread-like structures found within the nucleus of cells. Each chromosome contains many genes, and the entire set of an organism's genes is called its genome.

Moving on, heredity, or the passing of traits from parents to offspring, is a central focus of genetics. Here, traits can be physical, such as eye color or height, or biochemical, such as blood type or susceptibility to certain diseases.

The transmission of traits is governed by the principles of inheritance, which were first discovered by Gregor Mendel in the 19th century through his experiments with pea plants.

Mendel's laws of inheritance, including the law of segregation and the law of independent assortment, laid the foundation for how traits are passed from parents to offspring (modern genetics).

Genetics also explores how genetic information is transmitted and expressed in cells. Processes such as DNA replication, transcription, and translation are essential for making proteins and controlling gene expression.

Mutations, which are changes in the DNA sequence, can occur naturally or be caused by external factors like radiation or chemicals. So, understanding how mutations affect genes and traits is important in genetics.

In addition to studying traits within populations, genetics examines variation between individuals and species. This variation arises from genetic differences, environmental factors, and interactions between genes and the environment.

By studying patterns of genetic variation, scientists can learn about evolution, population genetics, and the genetic basis of diseases.

Genetics also plays a critical role in many fields, including medicine, agriculture, and biotechnology. In medicine, genetic research has led to significant advances in the diagnosis, treatment, and prevention of genetic disorders and common diseases.

In agriculture, genetics is used to improve crop yields, develop disease-resistant plants, and breed animals with desirable traits. In biotechnology, genetic engineering techniques are employed to produce pharmaceuticals, genetically modified organisms, and other products with applications in industry and medicine.

➤ Inheritance Patterns

In genetics, Inheritance patterns refer to the ways in which traits are passed from parents to offspring. These patterns are governed by the principles of genetics and can vary depending on the type of trait and the genetic makeup of the parents.

One of the most well-known inheritance patterns is Mendelian inheritance, which follows the laws discovered by Gregor Mendel through his experiments with pea plants in the 19th century.

Mendel's laws include the law of segregation, which states that each individual carries two copies of each gene, but only one copy is passed on to each offspring. Next, the law of independent assortment states that alleles for different traits are passed on independently of each other.

Mendelian inheritance patterns include dominant and recessive traits. Dominant traits are expressed when an individual has at least one dominant allele, while recessive traits are only expressed when an individual has two copies of the recessive allele.

For example, in Mendelian inheritance, the inheritance of traits like widow's peak hairline, attached earlobes, and tongue rolling follows simple dominant-recessive patterns.

In addition to Mendelian inheritance, there are other patterns of inheritance, such as incomplete dominance, monohybrid and dihybrid inheritance, codominance, and sex-linked inheritance. These will be discussed with more details.

- **Monohybrid Inheritance:**

Monohybrid inheritance falls under the broader category of Mendelian inheritance patterns. Specifically, it refers to the inheritance of a single gene with two contrasting alleles from one generation to the next.

This concept was first elucidated by Gregor Mendel in his experiments with pea plants where he observed the segregation of traits such as seed shape, seed color, and flower color.

In monohybrid inheritance, individuals inherit one allele from each parent for a specific trait. These alleles may be either dominant or recessive. The dominant allele masks the expression of the recessive allele when present in the genotype. However, if an individual inherits two copies of the recessive allele, the recessive trait is expressed in the phenotype.

For example, consider the inheritance of flower color in pea plants. Suppose there are two alleles for flower color: one for purple flowers (dominant allele, represented by "P") and one for white flowers (recessive allele, represented by "p").

A plant with genotype "PP" or "Pp" will have purple flowers, as the dominant allele masks the expression of the recessive allele. Only plants with genotype "pp" will exhibit white flowers, as there are no dominant alleles present to suppress the expression of the recessive allele.

Monohybrid inheritance patterns follow Mendel's laws of segregation and independent assortment. The law of segregation states that alleles segregate randomly during gamete formation, with each gamete receiving one allele for a particular trait.

The law of independent assortment dictates that alleles for different traits segregate independently of each other, resulting in the random assortment of alleles into gametes.

This inheritance pattern provides a foundational understanding of genetic transmission and serves as a basis for more complex inheritance patterns, such as dihybrid and trihybrid inheritance, where multiple traits are considered simultaneously. It is a fundamental concept in genetics and is applicable across various organisms, including plants, animals, and humans.

- **Dihybrid Inheritance:**

This refers to the inheritance of two different genes, each with two alleles, from one generation to the next. This concept was also elucidated by Gregor Mendel in his experiments with pea plants.

In dihybrid inheritance, individuals inherit alleles for two different traits and they are located on different gene loci and from each parent.

These alleles segregate independently during gamete formation, following Mendel's law of independent assortment. As a result, offspring inherit a combination of alleles for both traits which leads to a wide range of possible genetic combinations.

For example, consider the inheritance of seed color and seed shape in pea plants. Suppose there are two alleles for seed color: one for yellow seeds (dominant allele, represented by "Y") and one for green seeds (recessive allele, represented by "y").

Similarly, there are two alleles for seed shape: one for round seeds (dominant allele, represented by "R") and one for wrinkled seeds (recessive allele, represented by "r").

In a dihybrid cross between two pea plants that are heterozygous for both traits (YyRr x YyRr), the resulting offspring can exhibit various combinations of seed color and shape.

Through independent assortment, the alleles for seed color segregate independently of the alleles for seed shape, resulting in a 9:3:3:1 phenotypic ratio in the offspring.

Dihybrid inheritance provides insights into the inheritance of multiple traits simultaneously and as a fundamental concept in genetics, it deepens the understanding of genetic diversity, inheritance patterns, and genetic inheritance in complex organisms.

- **Incomplete Dominance:**

Incomplete dominance falls under the broader category of non-Mendelian inheritance patterns which deviate from the simple dominant-recessive relationship observed in Mendelian genetics.

In incomplete dominance, neither allele is completely dominant over the other. This results in a blending of traits in heterozygous individuals.

In incomplete dominance, the phenotype of heterozygous individuals is an intermediate or blend of the phenotypes associated with each allele. This contrasts with complete dominance, where the phenotype of heterozygous individuals is indistinguishable from that of homozygous dominant individuals.

An example of incomplete dominance can be seen in flower color in snapdragons. Suppose there are two alleles for flower color: one for red flowers (allele symbolized as "R") and one for white flowers (allele symbolized as "W"). In incomplete dominance, the heterozygous genotype (RW) results in pink flowers, which exhibit an intermediate phenotype between red and white.

Incomplete dominance challenges the traditional view of genetic dominance and underscores the complexity of gene expression and phenotype determination.

It is an important concept in genetics, providing insights into patterns of inheritance and genetic variation beyond the simple dominant-recessive model described by Mendel.

- **Codominance:**

Codominance is another type of non-Mendelian inheritance pattern where both alleles in a heterozygous individual are fully expressed, resulting in a phenotype that shows the traits of both alleles distinctly rather than blending them.

In codominance, neither allele is dominant or recessive over the other, and both are expressed simultaneously.

A classic example of codominance is seen in the ABO blood group system in humans. In this system, there are three alleles for the gene that determines blood type: IA, IB, and i. Alleles IA and IB are codominant, while allele i is recessive.

Individuals with genotype IAIA or IAi have blood type A, individuals with genotype IBIB or IBi have blood type B, and individuals with genotype IAIB have blood type AB. Here, both alleles IA and IB are expressed equally, resulting in the phenotype AB blood type, which shows traits of both A and B blood types.

Codominance provides another layer of complexity to genetic inheritance and contributes to the diversity of traits observed in populations. It highlights the notion that genetic variation can manifest in various ways, beyond the simple dominant-recessive relationship described by Mendel.

- **Sex-Linked Inheritance:**

Sex-linked inheritance refers to the inheritance patterns of genes located on the sex chromosomes, particularly the X chromosome in humans. Since males have one X and one Y chromosome (XY), and females have two X chromosomes (XX), sex-linked traits are typically more commonly expressed in males.

This is because males have only one copy of the X chromosome, and any recessive allele on the X chromosome will be expressed in the phenotype since there is no corresponding allele on the Y chromosome to mask it.

One of the most well-known examples of sex-linked inheritance is color blindness, a condition where individuals have difficulty distinguishing between certain colors.

The gene responsible for color blindness is located on the X chromosome, making it more common in males. In this case, if a male inherits the recessive allele for color blindness from his mother, he will be color blind because he has only one X chromosome.

However, females need to inherit two copies of the recessive allele to express the trait, making them less likely to be color blind.

Other examples of sex-linked traits include hemophilia, a bleeding disorder, and Duchenne muscular dystrophy, a progressive muscle disorder. Both of these conditions are caused by mutations in genes located on the X chromosome and primarily affect males.

Sex-linked inheritance follows different patterns compared to autosomal inheritance, where genes are located on non-sex chromosomes.

Understanding sex-linked inheritance is important in genetic counseling, diagnosis, and treatment of genetic disorders, especially those that disproportionately affect males due to their inheritance patterns.

➤ The Structure of DNA

The structure of DNA, or deoxyribonucleic acid, is a remarkable molecule that carries the genetic instructions necessary for the growth, development, functioning, and reproduction of all living organisms.

It is important to understand DNA because its intricate structure is fundamental to comprehending how genetic information is encoded, stored, and transmitted from one generation to the next.

- **Discovery of the Double Helix:**
  The structure of DNA was discovered by James Watson and Francis Crick in 1953, based on X-ray diffraction data obtained by Rosalind Franklin and Maurice Wilkins.
  Their model, known as the double helix, depicts two long DNA strands coiled around each other in a spiral staircase-like arrangement, forming a double helix or a twisted ladder.

- **Composition of DNA:** DNA is composed of nucleotides, which are the building blocks of the molecule. Each nucleotide consists of three components: a sugar molecule (deoxyribose), a phosphate group, and a nitrogenous base. The four nitrogenous bases found in DNA are adenine (A), thymine (T), cytosine (C), and guanine (G).

These bases pair specifically with each other: adenine pairs with thymine, and cytosine pairs with guanine. This complementary base pairing forms the rungs of the DNA ladder, with hydrogen bonds holding the base pairs together.

- **Double Helix Structure:** The sugar-phosphate backbones of the two strands run in opposite directions, with one strand oriented in the 5' to 3' direction and the other in the 3' to 5' direction.

  This antiparallel arrangement allows for the complementary base pairing between the nitrogenous bases. The arrangement of these base pairs along the DNA strands forms the genetic code, encoding the instructions for the synthesis of proteins and the regulation of cellular processes.

- **Advantages of the Double Helix Structure:** The double helix structure of DNA provides several key advantages. Firstly, it ensures the stability of the molecule, protecting the genetic information encoded within it.

  Secondly, the uniform diameter of the helix allows for efficient packaging of DNA into chromosomes, facilitating the orderly distribution of genetic material during cell division.

  Thirdly, the specific base pairing between adenine and thymine, and between cytosine and guanine, ensures the accurate replication of DNA during cell division, maintaining the integrity of the genetic code across generations.

- **Dynamic Nature of DNA:** The structure of DNA is dynamic and subject to various enzymatic processes. Enzymes such as DNA polymerase are responsible for replicating the DNA molecule during cell division, ensuring accurate transmission of genetic information to offspring. Additionally, DNA repair mechanisms exist to correct errors and maintain the integrity of the genetic code.

- **Role in Gene Expression:** In addition to its role as a storage molecule for genetic information, DNA is also the template for the synthesis of RNA (ribonucleic acid) and ultimately proteins.

  This process, known as gene expression, involves the transcription of DNA into RNA and the translation of RNA into proteins. The structure of DNA plays a critical role in regulating gene expression, as specific sequences of DNA serve as binding sites for regulatory proteins that control the activity of genes.

➤ The Mechanisms of Gene Expression and Regulation

Gene expression is the process by which the genetic information stored in DNA is used to direct the synthesis of proteins, which are the molecular machines that carry out most cellular functions.

Gene expression is tightly regulated to ensure that the right genes are expressed at the right time and in the right amount, allowing cells to respond to changing environmental conditions and developmental cues.

The process of gene expression begins with transcription, during which the DNA sequence of a gene is copied into a complementary RNA molecule called messenger RNA (mRNA).

This process is carried out by an enzyme called RNA polymerase, which binds to the DNA at a specific region called the promoter and unwinds the DNA double helix to expose the coding region of the gene.

RNA polymerase then adds complementary RNA nucleotides to the growing mRNA strand, following the base pairing rules (A-U and C-G in RNA). Once transcription is complete, the mRNA molecule is processed and transported out of the nucleus into the cytoplasm, where it serves as the template for protein synthesis.

In the cytoplasm, the mRNA molecule binds to ribosomes, which are the cellular machinery responsible for translating the genetic code into proteins.

Translation begins with the initiation phase, during which the ribosome assembles around the mRNA and identifies the start codon (usually AUG), signaling the beginning of protein synthesis.

Then, transfer RNA (tRNA) molecules carrying amino acids bind to complementary codons on the mRNA, bringing the appropriate amino acids into position to be linked together to form a polypeptide chain.

This process continues until a stop codon is reached, signaling the termination of protein synthesis and the release of the completed protein. The process of gene expression is tightly regulated at multiple levels to ensure that the right genes are expressed at the right time and in the right amounts.

Regulation can occur at the transcriptional level, where the activity of RNA polymerase is controlled by regulatory proteins that bind to specific DNA sequences near the promoter region of target genes. These regulatory proteins can either enhance or inhibit transcription, thereby modulating the expression of target genes.

In addition to transcriptional regulation, gene expression can also be regulated at the post-transcriptional level, where mRNA stability and translation efficiency are controlled by factors such as RNA-binding proteins and microRNAs (miRNAs).

These regulatory molecules can bind to specific sequences in the mRNA molecule and either promote or inhibit its translation into protein.
Furthermore, gene expression can be regulated at the post-translational level, where the activity and stability of proteins are controlled by processes such as protein modification (e.g., phosphorylation, glycosylation) and degradation. These modifications can alter the function and localization of proteins, allowing cells to rapidly respond to changes in their environment.

Overall, the mechanisms of gene expression and regulation are complex and highly coordinated processes that allow cells to precisely control their gene expression patterns in response to internal and external cues.

Evolutionary Theory: The Principles of Evolution by Natural Selection and Adaptation, and How It Explains The Diversity of Life on Earth.

Evolutionary theory is a fundamental concept in biology that explains the diversity of life on Earth and the processes by which organisms have changed and adapted over time.

It centrals on several key principles such as natural selection, adaptation, and the concept of common ancestry, which together provide a framework for understanding the origins and evolution of species.

One of the central tenets of evolutionary theory is natural selection, proposed by Charles Darwin in the 19th century. Natural selection operates on the idea that within any population, there is variation in traits among individuals.

Some of these variations are advantageous and they confer a greater likelihood of survival and reproduction in a given environment while others may be detrimental. Individuals with advantageous traits are more likely to survive and pass on their genes to the next generation, thereby increasing the frequency of those traits in the population over time.
This process leads to the gradual accumulation of adaptive traits within populations, ultimately resulting in the emergence of new species and the diversification of life forms.

Adaptation is another key concept in evolutionary theory, referring to the process by which organisms develop traits that enhance their survival and reproduction in their environment.

These traits can include physical features, behaviors, and physiological mechanisms that improve an organism's ability to obtain resources, avoid predators, and successfully reproduce.

Adaptations can arise through natural selection, as individuals with advantageous traits have a higher likelihood of surviving and passing on their genes. Over time, these adaptations can lead to the specialization of organisms to their particular ecological niches, resulting in the diversity of life observed on Earth.

The concept of common ancestry, or the idea that all living organisms are descended from a common ancestor, is also central to evolutionary theory.

This idea is supported by evidence from comparative anatomy, embryology, molecular biology, and the fossil record, which collectively provide insights into the relationships between different species and the patterns of descent and divergence over time.

By reconstructing the evolutionary history of species, scientists can infer the ancestral relationships between organisms and trace the origins of key traits and characteristics.

The evolutionary theory has profound implications for our understanding of the natural world and our place within it. It provides a unifying framework for biology that integrates diverse fields such as genetics, ecology, paleontology, and anthropology into a coherent narrative of life's history.

By expanding the processes of adaptation, speciation, and extinction, evolutionary theory also sheds light on the mechanisms driving biodiversity and ecosystem dynamics.

These principles of evolutionary theory have practical applications in fields such as medicine, agriculture, and conservation, informing strategies for disease prevention, crop improvement, and biodiversity conservation.

- **The Principles of Evolution by Natural Selection:**

Natural selection is an important principle of evolutionary theory that explains how organisms evolve and adapt to their environments over time. This principle was proposed by Charles Darwin in the 19th century and refined through subsequent research.

Natural selection is the process by which organisms with advantageous traits are more likely to survive and reproduce, while those with less favorable traits are less likely to pass on their genes to the next generation.

This differential reproductive success leads to the gradual accumulation of more advantageous traits within a population. This of course drives evolutionary change. The concept of natural selection rests on four key components. They are:

→ **Variation:** This states that within any population of organisms exists genetic variation. Meaning that individuals within the population differ from one another in terms of their traits.

These variations can be inherited from parents or arise through mutation, genetic recombination, or other processes.

Variation provides the raw material upon which natural selection acts, as it creates differences in traits that can affect an organism's ability to survive and reproduce.

→ **Differential Reproduction:** Natural selection also operates through the differential reproductive success of individuals with different traits as organisms that possess traits that are better suited to their environment are more likely to survive and reproduce, as well as pass on their advantageous traits to their offspring.

In contrast, individuals with less advantageous traits are less likely to survive and reproduce, leading to a decrease in the frequency of those traits within the population over time.

→ **Adaptation:** Over successive generations, natural selection leads to the accumulation of advantageous traits within a population, resulting in adaptations that improve an organism's fitness, or its ability to survive and reproduce in its environment.

Adaptations can take many forms, including physical features, behaviors, or physiological mechanisms that enhance an organism's chances of survival and reproductive success.

For example, the development of camouflage in prey species can increase their chances of avoiding predation, while the evolution of antibiotic resistance in bacteria enables them to survive exposure to antimicrobial drugs.

→ **Environmental Change:** Natural selection is also influenced by changes in the environment, including factors such as climate, habitat, food availability, predation pressure, and competition for resources.

Environmental changes can create new selective pressures that favor certain traits over others, leading to shifts in the frequency of traits within a population.

Organisms that are well-adapted to their current environment may become less fit if conditions change, highlighting the dynamic nature of natural selection.

Overall, natural selection is a powerful mechanism driving evolutionary change, shaping the diversity of life on Earth and leading to the remarkable adaptations observed in living organisms.

It provides a framework for understanding how species evolve in response to their environments and how complex traits and behaviors arise through the gradual accumulation of advantageous variations.

Now, by studying natural selection, scientists can gain insights into the processes of adaptation, speciation, and extinction, advancing our understanding of the natural world and our place within it.

- **The Principles of Evolution by Adaptation**

The principle of adaptation is a fundamental concept in biology and it highlights how organisms evolve traits that enhance their survival and reproduction in their respective environments.

Adaptation is driven by the process of natural selectio and it is a situation where individuals with advantageous traits are more likely to thrive and pass on their genes to subsequent generations. At its core, adaptation reflects the remarkable ability of organisms to adjust to their surroundings and exploit available resources effectively.

These adaptations can manifest in various forms such as physical features, behaviors, or physiological mechanisms, all geared towards improving an organism's fitness—their ability to survive and reproduce in their environment.

Physical adaptations are perhaps the most recognizable manifestations of adaptation. They include structural features such as camouflage, mimicry, or protective armor. These enable organisms to evade predators or enhance their hunting prowess.
A good example is the camouflage patterns of certain animals allow them to blend seamlessly into their surroundings, which effectively conceals them from predators or prey.

Behavioral adaptations involve changes in an organism's actions or habits to better suit their environment. Examples include migration, hibernation, or social behaviors like cooperation or territoriality.

Migration allows animals to move to more favorable habitats seasonally, while **hibernation** conserves energy during periods of resource scarcity. **Social behaviors**, such as cooperative hunting or parental care improves the survival chances of individuals within a group.

These physiological adaptations occur at the cellular or biochemical level and they enable organisms to cope with environmental challenges or exploit specific resources more efficiently. These adaptations could involve changes in metabolic processes, detoxification mechanisms, or tolerance to extreme conditions.

For instance, desert plants exhibit physiological adaptations such as water-conserving mechanisms or specialized photosynthetic pathways to thrive in arid environments.

Adaptation is not a static process but rather an ongoing response to changing environmental conditions. As environments evolve or shift, organisms must continually adapt to maintain their fitness and ensure their survival. Moreover, adaptation is context-dependent, with traits that confer advantages in one environment potentially becoming liabilities in another.

- **How These Principles Explain The Diversity of Life on Earth**

The principles of natural selection and adaptation are key to explaining the incredible variety of life on our planet. Natural selection acts like a filter, favoring organisms with traits that help them survive and reproduce.

Over time, this leads to the accumulation of helpful traits within populations thereby driving evolution. Adaptation is another big player. It lets organisms thrive in different environments by developing features or behaviors that suit their surroundings.

Think of animals with thick fur in cold climates or plants that conserve water in deserts. These adaptations help them survive and pass on their traits. Together, natural selection and adaptation shape the diversity of life on earth.

They drive the evolution of new species and enable organisms to thrive in all kinds of habitats, from icy tundras to steamy rainforests. These processes make our world so rich and varied.

Applying Scientific Knowledge: How To Think Critically About Scientific Concepts

Applying scientific knowledge means using critical thinking to understand and analyze scientific ideas. It involves looking at data, drawing conclusions based on evidence, and thinking logically. Now, for you to think critically about scientific concepts, you'll need these key steps:

- **Questioning:** Always ask questions about the scientific concepts you encounter. What evidence supports this idea? Are there alternative explanations? What are the limitations or uncertainties?

- **Evidence Evaluation:** Evaluate the evidence presented for scientific claims. Is it based on reliable data and sound experimental design? Are there biases or confounding factors that could affect the interpretation of results?

- **Analysis:** Analyze the data and information available to you. Look for patterns, trends, and inconsistencies. Consider how the evidence fits together to support or refute a hypothesis.

- **Integration:** Integrate new information with your existing knowledge base. How does this concept relate to what you already know? Does it challenge or reinforce your understanding of related topics?

- **Critical Thinking:** Apply critical thinking skills to evaluate arguments and draw logical conclusions. Consider the strengths and weaknesses of different viewpoints and assess the validity of scientific claims.

- **Skepticism**: Maintain a healthy skepticism towards scientific claims, particularly those that seem too good to be true or lack sufficient evidence. Remember that science is a process of inquiry and refinement, and no idea is beyond questioning.

- **Open-mindedness:** Remain open to new ideas and perspectives, even if they challenge your preconceived notions. Science is constantly evolving, and being open-minded allows you to adapt to new information and revise your understanding accordingly.

By applying these principles, you can develop a more critical and better understanding of scientific concepts that will enable you to engage with scientific information more effectively and make informed decisions based on evidence.

(Action Steps)
Anatomy Exercises and Quizzes Relevant to The TEAS 7 Exam

After reading through the anatomy topics, here are 35 questions prepared for you to answer correctly in the various TEAS 7 examination question format.

Multiple Choice Questions:
1. Which bone in the human body is commonly referred to as the "collarbone"?
   - A) Humerus
   - B) Scapula

- C) Clavicle
- D) Radius

2. What is the main function of the respiratory system?
    - A) Pumping blood to the heart
    - B) Digesting food
    - C) Exchanging gases between the body and the environment
    - D) Filtering toxins from the blood

Multiple Select Questions:

3. Which of the following are functions of the liver? (Select all that apply)
    - A) Producing bile
    - B) Storing glucose
    - C) Detoxifying harmful substances
    - D) Filtering lymph

4. Which of the following are types of muscle tissue found in the human body? (Select all that apply)
    - A) Skeletal muscle
    - B) Cardiac muscle
    - C) Smooth muscle
    - D) Adipose tissue

Supply the Answer:

5. Describe the process of bone remodeling and its importance for bone health.

Complete the Sentence:

6. The _____ system is responsible for regulating the body's metabolism and energy production.

Ordered Response:

7. Put the following steps of the cardiac cycle in the correct order:
    - A) Ventricular contraction (systole)

- B) Atrial contraction (atrial systole)
- C) Ventricular relaxation (diastole)

Multiple Choice Questions:

8. Which organ is responsible for filtering waste products from the blood and producing urine?
    - A) Liver
    - B) Kidney
    - C) Pancreas
    - D) Spleen
9. What is the function of the cerebrum in the brain?
    - A) Regulation of body temperature
    - B) Coordination of movement
    - C) Memory storage and higher cognitive functions
    - D) Regulation of heart rate

Multiple Select Questions:

10. Which of the following are components of the central nervous system? (Select all that apply)
    - A) Brain
    - B) Spinal cord
    - C) Peripheral nerves
    - D) Cranial nerves
11. Which of the following are functions of the digestive system? (Select all that apply)
    - A) Regulation of body temperature
    - B) Absorption of nutrients
    - C) Production of hormones
    - D) Elimination of waste

Supply the Answer:

12. Explain the role of neurotransmitters in transmitting signals between neurons.

Complete the Sentence:

13. The _____ system is responsible for protecting the body from pathogens and foreign invaders.

Ordered Response:

14. Put the following steps of muscle contraction in the correct order:
   - A) Calcium ions bind to troponin
   - B) Cross-bridge formation occurs
   - C) Myosin heads bind to actin filaments

Multiple Choice Questions:

15. Which part of the human brain is responsible for regulating basic bodily functions such as breathing and heart rate?
   - A) Cerebrum
   - B) Cerebellum
   - C) Medulla oblongata
   - D) Thalamus

16. What is the function of the lymphatic system in the human body?
   - A) Transportation of oxygen to cells
   - B) Regulation of body temperature
   - C) Defense against pathogens and diseases
   - D) Digestion of food

Multiple Select Questions:

17. Which of the following are functions of the skeletal system? (Select all that apply)
   - A) Protection of internal organs
   - B) Production of red blood cells
   - C) Storage of minerals such as calcium and phosphorus
   - D) Regulation of blood sugar levels

18. Which of the following are types of neurons found in the nervous system? (Select all that apply)

- A) Sensory neurons
- B) Motor neurons
- C) Interneurons
- D) Epithelial neurons

Supply the Answer:
19. Describe the process of synaptic transmission and how it facilitates communication between neurons.

Complete the Sentence:
20. The _____ system is responsible for supporting and protecting the body, as well as providing a framework for movement.

Ordered Response:
21. Put the following steps of the digestive process in the correct order:
- A) Absorption of nutrients in the small intestine
- B) Mechanical digestion in the mouth
- C) Chemical digestion in the stomach

Multiple Choice Questions:
22. Which of the following is NOT a function of the respiratory system?
- A) Exchange of gases
- B) Regulation of blood pH
- C) Production of hormones
- D) Vocalization
23. Which organ is responsible for filtering and detoxifying blood in the human body?
- A) Liver
- B) Kidney
- C) Spleen
- D) Pancreas

Multiple Select Questions:

24. Which of the following are components of the central nervous system? (Select all that apply)
- A) Brain
- B) Spinal cord
- C) Peripheral nerves
- D) Cranial nerves

25. Which of the following are functions of the muscular system? (Select all that apply)
- A) Production of heat
- B) Generation of movement
- C) Synthesis of hormones
- D) Maintenance of posture

Supply the Answer:
26. Explain the process of urine formation in the kidneys, including filtration, reabsorption, and secretion.

Complete the Sentence:
27. The _____ system is responsible for coordinating communication between different parts of the body through electrical signals.

Ordered Response:
28. Arrange the following structures of the respiratory system in the order in which air passes through them during inhalation:
- A) Trachea
- B) Bronchioles
- C) Alveoli

Multiple Choice Questions:
29. Which organ is responsible for the production of bile, essential for digestion?
- A) Pancreas

- B) Gallbladder
- C) Liver
- D) Stomach

30. Which of the following bones is classified as a long bone?
    - A) Vertebra
    - B) Sternum
    - C) Radius
    - D) Patella

Multiple Select Questions:

31. Which of the following are functions of the liver? (Select all that apply)
    - A) Synthesis of bile
    - B) Detoxification of harmful substances
    - C) Storage of urine
    - D) Regulation of blood glucose levels

32. Which of the following are types of muscle tissue found in the human body? (Select all that apply)
    - A) Skeletal muscle
    - B) Cardiac muscle
    - C) Adipose tissue
    - D) Smooth muscle

Supply the Answer:

33. Describe the structure of a typical long bone, including its main components and functions.

Complete the Sentence:

34. The _____ is responsible for regulating the body's internal environment and maintaining homeostasis.

Ordered Response:

35. Arrange the following stages of bone development in the correct sequence:
  - A) Ossification
  - B) Remodeling
  - C) Growth

Physiology Exercises and Quizzes Relevant to The TEAS 7 Exam

After reading through the Physiology topics, here are 35 questions prepared for you to answer correctly in the various TEAS 7 examination question format.

Multiple Choice:
1. What is the primary function of the hypothalamus?
  - A) Regulation of body temperature
  - B) Production of red blood cells
  - C) Regulation of blood glucose levels
  - D) Synthesis of neurotransmitters
2. Which hormone is responsible for promoting water retention in the kidneys?
  - A) Aldosterone
  - B) Insulin
  - C) Thyroxine
  - D) Growth hormone
3. What is the primary function of the tympanic membrane (eardrum)?
  - A) Regulation of balance
  - B) Amplification of sound waves
  - C) Protection of the inner ear
  - D) Transmission of sound vibrations

4. Which structures are part of the central nervous system (CNS)?
  - A) Brain
  - B) Spinal cord
  - C) Peripheral nerves
  - D) Cerebellum
5. Which of the following are functions of the lymphatic system?
  - A) Removal of interstitial fluid
  - B) Transport of fats
  - C) Production of bile
  - D) Immune response

Complete the Sentence:
6. The process by which light is focused on the retina is called _____.

7. The hormone _____ is responsible for regulating calcium levels in the blood.

Ordered Response:
8. Arrange the following structures of the eye in the correct order through which light passes:
  - Cornea
  - Pupil
  - Lens
  - Retina
9. Put the following steps of muscle contraction in the correct order:
  - Excitation-contraction coupling
  - Cross-bridge formation
  - Calcium release from the sarcoplasmic reticulum
  - Sliding filament theory

Multiple Choice:

10. Which organ system is responsible for filtering blood and removing waste products?
- A) Cardiovascular system
- B) Respiratory system
- C) Urinary system
- D) Endocrine system

11. What is the primary function of the cerebellum?
- A) Regulation of body temperature
- B) Coordination of movement
- C) Production of hormones
- D) Regulation of blood pressure

Multiple Select:

12. Which components are involved in the process of blood clotting?
- A) Platelets
- B) Red blood cells
- C) Fibrinogen
- D) Calcium ions

13. Which of the following are functions of the integumentary system?
- A) Regulation of body temperature
- B) Protection against pathogens
- C) Synthesis of vitamin D
- D) Production of insulin

Complete the Sentence:

14. The process of converting glucose into pyruvate in the absence of oxygen is called _____.

15. The hormone _____ is responsible for stimulating uterine contractions during childbirth.

Ordered Response:

16. Arrange the following events of the cardiac cycle in the correct order:
    - Atrial systole
    - Ventricular systole
    - Atrial diastole
    - Ventricular diastole
17. Put the following steps of the action potential in neurons in order:
    - Depolarization
    - Repolarization
    - Hyperpolarization

Multiple Choice:
18. Which gland is responsible for producing melatonin?
    - A) Pituitary gland
    - B) Thyroid gland
    - C) Pineal gland
    - D) Adrenal gland

19. What is the primary function of the alveoli in the lungs?
    - A) Gas exchange
    - B) Filtration of blood
    - C) Production of mucus
    - D) Regulation of blood pH

Multiple Select:
20. Which components are involved in the process of digestion?
    - A) Salivary glands
    - B) Gallbladder
    - C) Pancreas
    - D) Small intestine
21. Which of the following are characteristics of type 1 diabetes mellitus?
    - A) Autoimmune destruction of pancreatic beta cells
    - B) Insulin resistance

- C) Onset typically occurs in childhood or adolescence
- D) Requires insulin therapy for management

Complete the Sentence:
22. The process of converting amino acids into glucose or fat is known as _____.

23. The _____ system is responsible for regulating fluid balance in the body.

Ordered Response:
24. Arrange the following events of the menstrual cycle in the correct order:
   - Menstruation
   - Proliferative phase
   - Secretory phase

25. Put the following steps of urine formation in the correct order:
   - Filtration
   - Reabsorption
   - Secretion

Multiple Choice:
26. Which organ system is responsible for producing and secreting digestive enzymes?
   - A) Respiratory system
   - B) Endocrine system
   - C) Digestive system
   - D) Reproductive system
27. What is the primary function of the pancreas?
   - A) Producing insulin and glucagon
   - B) Filtering blood
   - C) Synthesizing bile

- D) Regulating blood pressure

Multiple Select:

28. Which components are involved in the process of respiration?
    - A) Diaphragm
    - B) Pharynx
    - C) Bronchioles
    - D) Epiglottis

29. Which of the following are characteristics of the sympathetic nervous system?
    - A) Fight or flight response
    - B) Slowing heart rate
    - C) Dilating pupils
    - D) Increasing digestive activity

Complete the Sentence:

30. The hormone _____ is responsible for stimulating milk production in the mammary glands.

31. The process by which excess water and waste products are removed from the blood is known as _____.

Ordered Response:

32. Arrange the following events of the reflex arc in the correct order:
    - Sensory receptor detects stimulus
    - Sensory neuron transmits signal to spinal cord
    - Interneuron processes information
    - Motor neuron transmits response to effector

33. Put the following steps of muscle fiber contraction in the correct order:
    - Calcium binds to troponin
    - Troponin-tropomyosin complex shifts
    - Myosin binds to actin

- Cross-bridge cycling occurs

Multiple Choice:

34. Which organ system is responsible for producing and releasing hormones that regulate various bodily functions?
    - A) Digestive system
    - B) Endocrine system
    - C) Lymphatic system
    - D) Muscular system
35. What is the primary function of the spleen?
    - A) Production of red blood cells
    - B) Storage of bile
    - C) Filtering blood
    - D) Production of digestive enzymes

Chemistry Exercises and Quizzes Relevant to The TEAS 7 Exam

After reading through the Chemistry topics, here are 40 questions prepared for you to answer correctly in the various TEAS 7 examination question format.

Multiple Choice:

1. What determines the atomic number of an atom?
   - A) Number of neutrons
   - B) Number of protons
   - C) Number of electrons
   - D) Number of electron shells
2. Which subatomic particles are found in the nucleus of an atom?
   - A) Electrons
   - B) Neutrons
   - C) Protons
   - D) Isotopes
3. Which electron shell determines the chemical behavior of an atom?

- A) Valence shell
- B) Inner shell
- C) Principal shell
- D) Subshell

Multiple Select:
4. Which of the following rules govern the arrangement of electrons in electron shells?
   - A) Aufbau principle
   - B) Pauli exclusion principle
   - C) Hund's rule
   - D) Newton's law
5. Which elements are typically involved in forming hydrogen bonds?
   - A) Hydrogen
   - B) Oxygen
   - C) Nitrogen
   - D) Fluorine

Complete the Sentence:
6. The number of protons in the nucleus of an atom is also known as its _____.

7. The outermost shell of an atom, which determines its chemical behavior, is called the _____ shell.

Ordered Response:
8. Arrange the following types of chemical bonds in order of increasing strength:
   - Covalent, Ionic, Hydrogen

9. Put the following types of chemical reactions in order from simplest to most complex:
   - Synthesis, Decomposition, Double Replacement

Multiple Choice:

10. Which type of chemical bond involves the transfer of electrons from one atom to another?
    - A) Covalent bond
    - B) Ionic bond
    - C) Hydrogen bond
    - D) Metallic bond
11. What is the primary characteristic of a solution?
    - A) Heterogeneous composition
    - B) Contains only solids
    - C) Homogeneous composition
    - D) No solute-solvent interaction

Multiple Select:
12. Which factors influence the rate of a chemical reaction?
    - A) Temperature
    - B) Concentration of reactants
    - C) Presence of catalysts
    - D) Molecular weight of products
13. Which of the following are examples of chemical properties?
    - A) Melting point
    - B) Flammability
    - C) Density
    - D) Reactivity

Complete the Sentence:
14. In a double replacement reaction, ions in two compounds _____.

15. The property of a substance that describes its ability to react with other substances and undergo chemical changes is known as _____.

Ordered Response:
16. Arrange the following states of matter in order of increasing compressibility:
    - Solid, Liquid, Gas

17. Put the following types of organic molecules in order of complexity:
   - Carbohydrates, Proteins, Lipids

Multiple Choice:

18. Which type of chemical reaction involves the combination of two or more substances to form a single product?
   - A) Synthesis reaction
   - B) Decomposition reaction
   - C) Single replacement reaction
   - D) Double replacement reaction
19. What is the primary function of enzymes in biochemical reactions?
   - A) Inhibit reactions
   - B) Increase activation energy
   - C) Accelerate reactions
   - D) Change reaction equilibrium

Multiple Select:

20. Which factors affect the solubility of a solute in a solvent?
   - A) Temperature
   - B) Pressure
   - C) Particle size
   - D) Chemical composition of solute
21. Which elements are commonly found in organic molecules?
   - A) Carbon
   - B) Hydrogen
   - C) Oxygen
   - D) Sodium

Complete the Sentence:

22. The breakdown of a single compound into two or more simpler substances is characteristic of a _____ reaction.

23. _____ are the building blocks of proteins, consisting of a central carbon atom bonded to an amino group, a carboxyl group, a hydrogen atom, and a variable side chain.

Ordered Response:
24. Arrange the following types of chemical bonds in order of increasing polarity:
   - Nonpolar covalent, Polar covalent, Ionic

25. Put the following steps of a chemical reaction in order:
   - Reactants collide, Activation energy is overcome, New bonds form, Products are released

Multiple Choice:
26. Which type of chemical reaction involves the breakdown of a single compound into two or more simpler substances?
   - A) Synthesis reaction
   - B) Decomposition reaction
   - C) Single replacement reaction
   - D) Double replacement reaction
27. What is the primary function of hydrogen bonds in biological molecules?
   - A) Forming strong covalent bonds
   - B) Providing structural support
   - C) Facilitating specific molecular interactions
   - D) Enhancing solubility

Multiple Select:
28. Which factors affect the rate of a chemical reaction?
   - A) Surface area
   - B) Catalysts
   - C) Temperature
   - D) pH
29. Which functional groups are commonly found in organic molecules?
   - A) Hydroxyl (-OH)
   - B) Carboxyl (-COOH)

- C) Nitrate (-NO3)
- D) Sulfhydryl (-SH)

Complete the Sentence:

30. The formation of a bond between a metal and a nonmetal resulting in the transfer of electrons is characteristic of an _____ bond.

31. The property of a substance that describes its resistance to flow is known as _____.

Ordered Response:

32. Arrange the following states of matter in order of increasing kinetic energy:
   - Solid, Liquid, Gas

33. Put the following types of chemical reactions in order from most energy-releasing to least energy-releasing:
   - Combustion, Synthesis, Decomposition

Multiple Choice:

34. Which type of chemical bond involves the sharing of electrons between atoms?
   - A) Ionic bond
   - B) Covalent bond
   - C) Hydrogen bond
   - D) Metallic bond

35. What is the primary function of enzymes in biochemical reactions?
   - A) Inhibit reactions
   - B) Increase activation energy
   - C) Accelerate reactions
   - D) Change reaction equilibrium

Supply Answer:

36. Define the term "atomic number" and explain its significance in determining the identity of an atom.

37. Describe the process of hydrogen bonding and provide an example of its importance in biological systems.

38. Explain the difference between polar and nonpolar covalent bonds, and provide examples of molecules exhibiting each type of bond.

39. Discuss the role of enzymes in biochemical reactions, including how they increase reaction rates and their specificity for substrates.

40. Define the term "chemical reaction" and provide an example of a chemical reaction, including the chemical equation representing the reaction.

Biology Exercises and Quizzes Relevant to The TEAS 7 Exam

After reading through the Biology topics, here are 40 questions prepared for you to answer correctly in the various TEAS 7 examination question format.

Multiple Choice:
1. What is the primary function of the Golgi apparatus in a eukaryotic cell?
   - A) Energy production
   - B) Protein synthesis
   - C) Modification and packaging of proteins
   - D) DNA replication
2. Which organelle is responsible for breaking down cellular waste and damaged organelles?
   - A) Mitochondria
   - B) Endoplasmic reticulum
   - C) Golgi apparatus
   - D) Lysosomes

3. During which stage of mitosis do chromosomes align at the cell's equatorial plane?
   - A) Prophase
   - B) Metaphase
   - C) Anaphase
   - D) Telophase

Multiple Select:
4. Which organelles are involved in cellular respiration? (Select all that apply)
   - A) Mitochondria
   - B) Endoplasmic reticulum
   - C) Golgi apparatus
   - D) Chloroplasts

5. Which nitrogenous bases are found in DNA? (Select all that apply)
   - A) Adenine
   - B) Thymine
   - C) Cytosine
   - D) Uracil

Ordered Response:
6. Arrange the stages of mitosis in the correct order:
   - A) Telophase
   - B) Anaphase
   - C) Prophase
   - D) Metaphase

Complete the Sentence:
7. The primary function of the cytoplasm is to provide a medium for cellular activities and support organelles, including the endoplasmic reticulum, Golgi apparatus, mitochondria, and ribosomes, crucial for the cell's _____.

8. The endoplasmic reticulum plays a key role in protein synthesis and lipid metabolism, with the rough ER having ribosomes attached to its surface

involved in _____, while the smooth ER lacks ribosomes and is responsible for _____.

Supply Answer:

9. Discuss the role of the cytoskeleton in maintaining cell shape and facilitating cell movement.

10. Explain how mutations in DNA can affect gene expression and protein function, providing examples of genetic disorders caused by mutations.

Multiple Choice:

11. What is the function of chloroplasts in plant cells?
   - A) Cellular respiration
   - B) Protein synthesis
   - C) Photosynthesis
   - D) DNA replication

12. Which cellular organelle is responsible for processing and packaging proteins for secretion or delivery to other cellular locations?
   - A) Nucleus
   - B) Golgi apparatus
   - C) Lysosomes
   - D) Endoplasmic reticulum

13. During cellular respiration, where does the citric acid cycle (Krebs cycle) occur?
   - A) Mitochondria
   - B) Nucleus
   - C) Cytoplasm
   - D) Golgi apparatus

Multiple Select:

14. Which components are found in a nucleotide? (Select all that apply)
   - A) Phosphate group
   - B) Sugar molecule
   - C) Nitrogenous base
   - D) Amino acid

15. Which of the following are stages of the cell cycle? (Select all that apply)
  - A) Interphase
  - B) Mitosis
  - C) Cytokinesis
  - D) Replication

Ordered Response:
16. Arrange the steps of protein synthesis in the correct order:
  - A) Translation
  - B) Transcription
  - C) Replication
  - D) Folding

Complete the Sentence:
17. The primary function of mitochondria is to produce ATP through
_____.

18. The structure of DNA, known as the double helix, was discovered by
_____ in 1953.

Supply Answer:
19. Discuss the differences between prokaryotic and eukaryotic cells, highlighting their structural and functional distinctions.

20. Explain the significance of the genetic code in determining the sequence of amino acids during protein synthesis.

Multiple Choice:
21. During protein synthesis, which molecule carries the genetic information from the DNA in the nucleus to the ribosomes in the cytoplasm?
  - A) DNA polymerase
  - B) Transfer RNA (tRNA)
  - C) Messenger RNA (mRNA)
  - D) Ribosomal RNA (rRNA)

22. Which process involves the division of a diploid cell into two identical diploid daughter cells?
- A) Mitosis
- B) Meiosis
- C) Transcription
- D) Translation

Multiple Select:
23. Which molecules are involved in protein synthesis? (Select all that apply)
- A) mRNA
- B) tRNA
- C) rRNA
- D) DNA polymerase

Ordered Response:
24. Arrange the steps of cellular respiration in the correct sequence:
- A) Glycolysis
- B) Citric acid cycle (Krebs cycle)
- C) Electron transport chain
- D) Oxidative phosphorylation

Complete the Sentence:
25. The process of meiosis results in the formation of _____.

26. Enzymes catalyze chemical reactions by _____.

Multiple Select:
27. Which of the following are components of a nucleotide?
- A) Sugar molecule
- B) Phosphate group
- C) Nitrogenous base
- D) Amino acid

Complete the Sentence:

28. The process of cellular respiration involves the breakdown of glucose molecules to produce ATP through a series of _____ reactions.

Ordered Response:
29. Arrange the following stages of the cell cycle in the correct sequence:
   - A) G1 phase
   - B) S phase
   - C) G2 phase
   - D) Mitosis

Complete the Sentence:
30. The plasma membrane is composed of a _____ bilayer.

Multiple Choice:
31. What is one of the central tenets of evolutionary theory proposed by Charles Darwin?
   - A) Genetic variation
   - B) Genetic recombination
   - C) Environmental change
   - D) Natural selection

Multiple Select:
32. Which concepts are central to evolutionary theory? (Select all that apply)
   - A) Natural selection
   - B) Adaptation
   - C) Genetic mutation
   - D) Artificial selection

Ordered Response:
33. Arrange the following components of natural selection in the correct sequence:
   - A) Variation
   - B) Differential reproduction
   - C) Adaptation
   - D) Environmental change

Complete the Sentence:
34. Adaptation is a fundamental concept in biology that elucidates how organisms evolve traits that enhance their survival and reproduction in their respective _____.

Multiple Choice:
35. What is the primary implication of evolutionary theory for understanding the natural world?
   - A) Understanding species extinction
   - B) Integrating diverse fields of biology
   - C) Exploring artificial selection
   - D) Identifying genetic mutations

Multiple Select:
36. Which fields of study are integrated into a coherent narrative by evolutionary theory? (Select all that apply)
   - A) Genetics
   - B) Astronomy
   - C) Paleontology
   - D) Sociology

Ordered Response:
37. Arrange the following stages of natural selection in the correct sequence:
   - A) Genetic variation
   - B) Differential reproduction
   - C) Adaptation
   - D) Environmental change

Complete the Sentence:
38. Environmental change influences natural selection by creating new _____ that favor certain traits over others.

Multiple Choice:
39. What does adaptation allow organisms to do?

- A) Remain unchanged in their environment
- B) Evolve rapidly
- C) Thrive in different environments
- D) Resist genetic variation

Ordered Response:

40. Arrange the following concepts related to adaptation in the correct sequence:
    - A) Physical adaptations
    - B) Behavioral adaptations
    - C) Physiological adaptations
    - D) Adaptive responses to environmental changes

Chapter 6:

English Language Proficiency

Welcome to Chapter 6! In this chapter, we'll talk about the essential aspects of English language that you ought to master if you're aiming to ace your TEAS 7 examination. We'll start from grammar basics to sentence structure, spelling, punctuations, and even practical examples and exercises that will give you a deeper understanding and increase your proficiency in English Language.

English Language and Importance of English Language Proficiency for the TEAS

Your proficiency in English language is crucial for excelling in the TEAS examination. This is because the TEAS exam assesses your readiness for entry into nursing and any other health programs.

Now, your proficiency in English ensures clear communication, comprehension of exam questions, and effective expression of ideas in both written and verbal forms. Without a solid grasp of the English language basics, you may struggle to comprehend passages, answer questions accurately, and communicate effectively.

This will ultimately hinder your success in the TEAS exam and your future academic pursuits in nursing or any healthcare-related field. Therefore, mastering English language skills is imperative for achieving optimal performance on the TEAS exam and ensuring success in nursing and allied health education and careers.

Grammar and Sentence Structure

➢ Grammar

Grammar is like the rulebook for how we put together sentences in English. It covers things like how words are arranged, how sentences are structured, and even how to use punctuation.

It refers to the set of rules and principles that govern the structure, composition, and usage of language, particularly in the form of sentences and phrases.
It comprises of various aspects such as syntax (sentence structure), morphology (word formation), semantics (meaning), and grammar rules (e.g., verb conjugation, agreement, and punctuation).

In essence, grammar is the framework that helps you construct a sentence that makes sense and gets your point across clearly. These grammar rules helps improve your communication in both written and spoken English language.

Here is a detailed and easy-to-understand explanation of the various grammar rules existing in English language.

- **Rule 1- Subject-Verb Agreement**

Subject-verb agreement means that the subject and the verb in a sentence must match. It is a fundamental grammatical concept that ensures consistency between the subject (the person, thing, or idea that performs the action) and the verb (the action or state of being) in a sentence.

In English, verbs change form to match the number and person of the subject. So if the subject is one thing, the verb must be for one thing too. If the subject is more than one thing, the verb needs to be for more than one thing.

The Subject-Verb Agreement is broken into:

→ **Singular Subjects and Singular Verbs:** When the subject of a sentence is singular (referring to one person, thing, or idea), the verb must also be singular.
For example: "The cat **runs** quickly."
(Subject: **"cat"** - singular; Verb: **"runs"** - singular)

→ **Plural Subjects and Plural Verbs:** When the subject of a sentence is plural (referring to more than one person, thing, or idea), the verb must also be plural.
For example: "The cats **run** quickly."
(Subject: **"cats"** - plural; Verb: **"run"** - plural)

→ **Compound Subjects:** When a sentence has two or more subjects joined by **"and,"** the verb is usually plural. However, if the subjects are considered a single unit or refer to the same thing, a singular verb is used.

For example: "John **and** Mary **are** going to the store."
(Plural subjects)
"Bread and butter **is** my favorite breakfast." (Singular subject)

→ **Indefinite Pronouns:** Some indefinite pronouns, such as **"everyone," "nobody," "each," "either,"** and **"neither,"** are always singular. Others, like **"both," "many," "few," and "several,"** are always plural.

For example: "Everybody **wants** to succeed." (Singular subject)
"Many of the students **are** studying for the exam." (Plural subject)

→ **Collective Nouns:** Collective nouns refer to groups of people or things as a single entity and it can take either a singular or plural verb depending on context of the sentence. That is, if we see them as one unit, we use the one form of the verb. If we see them as many people, we use the many form of the verb.

For example:
"The team **is** playing well."
(Singular verb, treating the team as a single unit)
"The team **are** arguing among themselves."
(Plural verb, emphasizing the individuals within the team.)

→ **Special Cases:** There are some irregular verbs and unusual sentence structures that may require careful attention to subject-verb agreement.

For example:
"The news **is** shocking." (Singular verb, treating "news" as a singular concept)
- "Mathematics **is** my favorite subject." (Singular verb, treating "mathematics" as an abstract concept)

Rule 2: Verb Tenses (Present, Past, Future)

Verb tenses are used to indicate the time of an action or state of being. It tells you when an action happens. It could be in the present, the past, or the future. All these is to help you understand the timing of events in a sentence. In English, there are three primary verb tenses: present, past, and future. Each tense can be further divided into four aspects: simple, continuous (or progressive), perfect, and perfect continuous.

The difference between tense and aspect lies in how they express time and duration in relation to the action of a verb:

For Tense, it indicates the time when an action occurs (past, present, future). It answers the question "When does the action happen?" Examples of tenses include past tense (e.g., "I walked"), present tense (e.g., "I walk"), and future tense (e.g., "I will walk").

While Aspect indicates the duration, completion, or ongoing nature of an action. It provides additional information about the action's state or progress. Aspect answers the question "How is the action unfolding?" (completed, ongoing, repeated, etc.) Examples of aspects include simple aspect (e.g., "I walk"), continuous aspect (e.g., "I am walking"), perfect aspect (e.g., "I have walked"), and perfect continuous aspect (e.g., "I have been walking").

Now, let's dive into each tense and aspect:

Present Tense: This is used to talk about actions that are happening now or that happen regularly. This is formed by using the base form of the verb (e.g., "I eat," "She runs"). For example:
  - "She walks to school every day."
  - "He plays basketball on weekends."
  - "I eat breakfast at 8 AM."

Present Continuous: This type of tense indicates actions that are happening at the moment of speaking or ongoing actions. It is formed using the present tense of the verb "to be" (am/is/are) with the present participle (verb + -ing) (e.g., "I am eating," "She is running").

Past Tense: This is used to talk about actions that have already happened. That is, completed actions or events that occurred at a specific point in the past. Regular verbs form the past tense by adding -ed to the base form or word (e.g., "I walked," "She danced"), while irregular verbs forms unique past tense words (like "I went," "She ate").
Past Tense example:
  - "She walked to school yesterday."
  - "He played basketball last Saturday."
  - "I ate breakfast at 8 AM this morning."

Past Continuous: This indicates actions that were ongoing or in progress at a specific time in the past. It is formed by using the past tense of the verb "to be" (was/were) with the present participle (e.g., "I was studying," "She was sleeping").

Future Tense: This is used to talk about actions that will happen later, in the future. It is formed using the modal verb "will" or "shall" followed by the base form of the verb (e.g., "I will travel," "She shall call"). For example:
  - "She will walk to school tomorrow."
  - "He will play basketball next Saturday."
  - "I will eat breakfast at 8 AM tomorrow."

Future Continuous: This indicates actions that will be ongoing or in progress at a specific time in the future. It is formed using the future tense of the verb "to be" (will be/shall be) with the present participle (e.g., "I will be working," "She shall be studying").

Each tense can be further divided into different forms to show more specific timing or relationships between actions:

Simple Aspect: The simple aspect is used to describe actions that are singular, habitual, or general statements without emphasizing their ongoing nature, its duration or completion.

For Example:
- "She walks to school every day." (habitual action)
- "He plays basketball on weekends." (regular action)
- "I eat breakfast at 8 AM." (general truth or habitual action).

Continuous (Progressive) Aspect: This form indicates actions that are ongoing or in progress at a specific time. For example:
  - Present Continuous: "She is walking to school."
  - Past Continuous: "She was walking to school when it started raining."
  - Future Continuous: "She will be walking to school at 8 AM tomorrow."

Perfect Aspect: This form indicates actions that are completed or finished before a certain point in time. It is divided into:
  - Present Perfect: This describes actions that occurred at an indefinite time in the past or have relevance to the present moment. It is formed using the auxiliary verb "have" or "has" with the past participle of the main verb (e.g., "I have seen," "She has eaten").
  - Past Perfect: This indicates actions that were completed before a specific point in the past. It is formed using the past tense of the auxiliary verb "have" (had) with the past participle (e.g., "I had finished," "She had left").

Perfect Aspect example:
  - Present Perfect: "She has walked to school every day this week."
  - Past Perfect: "She had walked to school before it started raining."
  - Future Perfect: "She will have walked to school by the time you arrive."

Perfect Continuous Aspect:
  - Present Perfect Continuous: Expresses actions that began in the past and continue into the present or have just stopped. It is formed using the present perfect of the auxiliary verb "have" or "has" with "been" and the present participle (e.g., "I have been studying," "She has been working").

- Past Perfect Continuous: Describes actions that were ongoing for a period of time before another action or time in the past. It is formed using the past perfect of the auxiliary verb "have" (had) with "been" and the present participle (e.g., "I had been waiting," "She had been sleeping").

Rule 3: Pronoun Antecedent Agreement

Pronoun-antecedent agreement is a grammatical principle that ensures that pronouns (words like "he," "she," "it," "they," "them," etc.) agree in number, gender, and person with their antecedents (the words they refer to) in a sentence. This agreement helps to avoid confusion and maintain clarity in writing.

Example:
- Incorrect: "Each of the students brought their books to class." (Incorrect agreement)
- Correct: "Each of the students brought his or her book to class." (Correct agreement)

In this example, "each" is a singular subject, so the pronoun referring to it should also be singular. Using "their" instead of "his or her" creates a disagreement because "their" is plural, while "each" is singular.

Here's a detailed explanation of pronoun-antecedent agreement:

Number Agreement: Pronouns must agree with their antecedents in number. If the antecedent is singular, the pronoun must be singular. If the antecedent is plural, the pronoun must be plural.
For Example:
- Singular antecedent: "The student submitted **his** assignment."
  - Plural antecedent: "The students submitted **their** assignments."

Gender Agreement: Pronouns must agree with their antecedents in gender. This means using pronouns that match the gender of their antecedents. Also, it can be said that English traditionally lacks gender-neutral pronouns. However, efforts are made to use gender-neutral language where possible:
   - Example:
   - Masculine: "He brought his backpack." (Correct)
   - Feminine: "She brought her backpack." (Correct)
   - Neutral: "It brought its backpack." (Correct)

Person Agreement: Pronouns should match the person of their antecedents, whether first person (I, we), second person (you), or third person (he, she, it, they). Maintaining person agreement ensures consistency in the narrative perspective.
For Example:
   - First Person: "I brought my book." (Correct)
   - Second Person: "You brought your book." (Correct)
   - Third Person: "He brought his book." (Correct)

Ambiguous Antecedents: Ambiguity arises when it's unclear which noun a pronoun refers to. So avoid ambiguity by ensuring clear antecedents for pronouns else you'll cause confusion in the minds of your readers.
For example:
- Ambiguous: "Jane told Sarah that she should go home." (It's unclear who should go home—Jane or Sarah?)
   - Clear: "Jane told Sarah that Sarah should go home."

Indefinite Pronouns: Pronouns such as "everyone," "anyone," "each," and "everyone" are singular and require singular pronouns:
   - "Everyone brought **his** or **her** own lunch."

Collective Nouns: Collective nouns refer to groups of people or things. When referring to collective nouns like "team," "group," or "family," consider whether the collective noun is acting as a single unit or as individuals:
   - "The team celebrated **its** victory." (as a unit)
   - "The team members celebrated **their** victory." (as individuals)

Rule 4: Proper Use of Articles (a, an, the)

Articles are small words that precede nouns to provide information about the noun. In English, there are two types of articles: definite (the) and indefinite (a, an). Understanding the proper use of articles is essential for you to communicate clearly and accurately. Here's a more in-depth look at how to use articles correctly:

Definite Article "The":

"The" is known as the definite article because it refers to a specific noun that is known to both the speaker and the listener or reader. It is used before singular and plural nouns when the speaker wants to indicate a particular person, thing, or idea.

  - Examples:
   - "Please pass **the** salt." (Referring to a specific salt shaker that both the speaker and listener know about.)
   - "I saw **the** movie last night." (Referring to a specific movie that was watched.)

Indefinite Articles "A" and "An":

- "A" and "an" are known as indefinite articles because they refer to non-specific nouns. "A" is used before words that begin with a consonant sound. "An" is used before words that begin with a vowel sound. Both "a" and "an" are used to introduce a noun for the first time or to refer to any member of a group. These articles introduce non-specific or generic nouns.

  - Examples:
   - "I saw **a** cat in the garden." (Referring to any cat, not a specific one.)
   - "She ate **an** apple for breakfast." (Referring to any apple, not a specific one.)
   - "He bought **a** car." (Referring to any car, not a specific one.)
   - "She is an engineer." (Referring to her profession in a general sense.)

Zero Article:

Some nouns do not require an article. This is known as the zero article. Zero articles is also used before uncountable nouns used in a general sense.
  - Examples:
    - "Cats are mammals." (Referring to cats in general.)
    -"She loves music." (Not "She loves the music.")
    - "Water is essential for life." (Referring to water in general.)
    - "He likes to play basketball." (Referring to basketball as a general activity.)

Use of "The" with Superlatives and Ordinal Numbers:
"The" is used with superlative adjectives and ordinal numbers to refer to a specific item in a group.
  - Examples:
    - "She is **the** tallest girl in the class." (Referring to a specific girl who is the tallest among others.)
    - "He won **the** first prize in the competition." (Referring to a specific prize—the top prize.)

Use of "The" with Unique Nouns:
  - "The" is used with unique nouns that are one of a kind or well-known.
  - Examples:
    - "She is **the** President of the United States." (Referring to a specific office holder.)
    - "We visited **the** Eiffel Tower in Paris." (Referring to a specific landmark.)

Rule 5: The Correct Use of Prepositions

Prepositions are words that establish relationships between different elements within a sentence. They usually indicate location, time, direction, or other relationships between nouns, pronouns, or phrases in a sentence. Prepositions often come before nouns, pronouns, or gerunds (verbs ending in "-ing") to provide additional information about their relationship with other parts of the sentence.
Here's a detailed explanation of how to use prepositions effectively:

Location and Position:
Prepositions like "in," "on," and "at" are used to indicate location or position. "In" is used to denote being inside an enclosed space or within the boundaries of an area.

- Example: "The keys are in the drawer."

"On" is used to indicate being in contact with a surface or in a specific position.

- Example: "The book is on the table."

"At" is used to specify a precise location or position.

- Example: "We'll meet at the park entrance."

Other prepositions like "under," "beside," "between," and "among" indicate relative positions in relation to other objects. For example, "The cat is under the table," "She stood beside the car," "The ball is between the two chairs," and "He is among friends."

Time:
Prepositions like "in," "on," and "at" are also used to express time-related relationships.

"In" is used to refer to periods of time, such as months, years, seasons, or parts of the day.

- For example: "She was born in May."

"On" is used to specify particular days and dates.

- For example: "The meeting is on Monday." It indicates a specific point in time.

"At" is used to indicate specific times or moments.

- For example: "We'll meet at 9 o'clock."

- "Since" is used to indicate the starting point of a period of time. For example, "She has been studying since morning." It denotes the beginning of a duration.

- "For" is used to indicate the duration of an action or state. For example, "They have been friends for ten years." It specifies the length of time for which something has been happening.

Direction and Movement:
 - Prepositions like "to," "from," "into," and "out of" are used to indicate direction or movement.
"To" is used to show movement towards a destination. For example: "He walked to the store."
"From" is used to indicate the starting point of movement. For example: "She came from the airport."
"Into" is used to indicate movement towards the inside or interior of something. For example: "The cat jumped into the box."
"Onto" denotes movement to a position on a surface. For example, "She climbed onto the roof."
"Out of" is used to show movement away from the inside or interior of something. For example: "She took the cookies out of the jar."
"Toward(s)" specifies movement in the direction of something. For example, "She walked toward(s) the park."

Purpose and Function:
Prepositions like "for," "with," "without," "by," and "of" indicate the purpose or function of an action or object.
"For" denotes the intended purpose or beneficiary of an action. For example, "He bought flowers for his mother."
"With" indicates the instrument or means used to perform an action. For example, "She opened the door with a key."
"Without" indicates the absence of something. For example, "He ate dinner without dessert."
"By" specifies the agent or means by which an action is performed. For example, "The letter was written by Mary."
"Of" indicates possession, association, or content. For example, "The pages of the book," "The keys of the car," "A cup of tea."

Rule 6: Agreement in Number (Singular vs. Plural)

Agreement in number, whether singular or plural, refers to ensuring that the subject of a sentence matches the verb and other elements in terms of singular or plural form. This agreement helps maintain clarity and coherence in writing by ensuring that all components of a sentence are in harmony.

Singular vs. Plural:
Singular: Refers to one person, thing, or concept.
For example: The cat **is** sleeping. (The subject "cat" is singular, so the verb "is" is also singular.)
Plural: Refers to more than one person, thing, or concept.
For example: The cats **are** sleeping. (The subject "cats" is plural, so the verb "are" is also plural.)

Rules for Subject-Verb Agreement:

Singular Subject: When the subject is singular, the verb must be singular.
For example: The book **is** on the table.

Plural Subject: When the subject is plural, the verb must be plural.
For example: The books **are** on the table.

Compound Subjects: If two subjects are joined by "and," the verb is usually plural.
For example: Mary **and** John **are** going to the party.

Collective Nouns: A collective noun representing a group of individuals can take either a singular or plural verb, depending on the context.
For example: The team **is** practicing. (Singular)
For example: The team **are** wearing their uniforms. (Plural)

Indefinite Pronouns: Some indefinite pronouns, like "everyone," "anyone," and "each," are always singular and require singular verbs.
For example: Everyone **wants** to go.

Agreement with Quantifiers: Words that indicate quantity, like "some," "many," or "all," may take either a singular or plural verb, depending on the noun they modify.

For example: Some of the cake **has** been eaten. (Singular)
For example: Some of the cookies **have** been eaten. (Plural)

Rule 7: Adjective and Adverb Usage

Adjectives and adverbs are essential parts of speech in English gramma. They serve distinct functions in modifying nouns, pronouns, verbs, and other adjectives or adverbs. So it is very important to understand their usage for effectively describing and qualifying elements within sentences.

Adjective Usage:

Definition: Adjectives are words that modify or describe nouns or pronouns by providing more information about their qualities, characteristics, or attributes. They answer questions like "what kind?" "which one?" "how many?" or "how much?" For example, in the phrase "the **blue** sky," "blue" is the adjective describing the sky's color.

Placement of Adjectives: Adjectives typically precede the noun they modify in English sentences. They can also follow the verb "to be." Also, certain adjectives, like "enough," "plenty," "all," "some," and "any," can go before or after the noun.

For example: She wore a **beautiful** dress.

Types of Adjectives:

Descriptive Adjectives: These adjectives describe the physical or qualitative attributes of nouns, such as color, size, shape, etc. For example, in the phrase "a **large** house," "large" describes the size of the house.

Demonstrative Adjectives: These adjectives point out specific nouns and indicate their proximity in space or time. They answer the question "which one?"
Common examples include "this," "that," "these," and "those." For instance, in the phrase "I like **this** book," "this" points to a specific book.

Quantitative Adjectives: These express the quantity or amount of a noun. Examples include "many," "few," "some," "several," "all," "no," "each," and "every." For instance, in the phrase "**several** students," "several" indicates the quantity of students.

Proper Adjectives: These adjectives are derived from proper nouns and describe specific people, places, or things. They are capitalized. For example, in the phrase "an **Italian** restaurant," "Italian" describes the type of restaurant.

Possessive Adjectives: These show ownership or possession of a noun. Examples include "my," "your," "his," "her," "its," "our," and "their." For example, in the phrase "his **car**," "his" shows ownership of the car.

Adverb Usage:

Definition: Adverbs are words that modify or describe verbs, adjectives, other adverbs, or entire clauses by providing more information about manner, place, time, frequency, degree, or reason. They answer questions like "how?" "when?" "where?" "why?" or "to what extent?"
For example, in the phrase "she speaks **fluently**," "fluently" is the adverb describing how she speaks.

Placement of Adverbs: Adverbs can appear in different positions within a sentence, depending on the type of adverb and the context. They can be placed before or after the verb, before or after the adjective or adverb they modify, or at the beginning or end of a sentence for emphasis.

For example: She **quickly** ran. / She ran **quickly**.

Types of Adverbs:

Adverbs of Manner: These describe how an action is performed. Examples include "quickly," "slowly," "carefully," "well," and "badly." For instance, in the phrase "he drove **carefully**," "carefully" describes how he drove.

Adverbs of Place: These describe the location or position of an action. Examples include "here," "there," "everywhere," "near," "far," and "away." For instance, in the phrase "they went **away**," "away" indicates where they went.

Adverbs of Time: These adverbs indicate when an action occurs. Examples include "now," "soon," "today," "yesterday," "already," and "never." For example, in the phrase "she will leave **soon**," "soon" indicates when she will leave.

Adverbs of Frequency: These describe how often an action occurs. Examples include "always," "often," "sometimes," "rarely," "never," and "seldom." For example, in the phrase "he **always** arrives early," "always" indicates how often he arrives early.

Adverbs of Degree: These express the intensity or degree of an action or quality. Examples include "very," "too," "extremely," "quite," "almost," and "barely." For instance, in the phrase "she is **very** happy," "very" indicates the degree of happiness.

Rule 8: Use of Conjunctions (and, but, or, so)

Conjunctions are words that connect words, phrases, or clauses within a sentence. They help to establish relationships between different parts of a sentence, such as joining similar ideas, contrasting ideas, or indicating cause and effect. Common conjunctions include "and," "but," "or," "so," "yet," "for," "nor," and "although."

Types of Conjunctions:
There are different types of conjunctions and they include:

Coordinating Conjunctions: These conjunctions join words, phrases, or independent clauses of equal importance within a sentence. The most common coordinating conjunctions are "and," "but," "or," "so," "yet," and "for." For example:
 - "I like coffee **and** tea." (connects two similar items)
 - "He studied hard **but** didn't pass the exam." (expressing contrast)

Subordinating Conjunctions: These conjunctions join a subordinate (dependent) clause to a main (independent) clause inorder to create complex sentences. They indicates a relationship of time, place, cause, condition, or concession. Examples of subordinating conjunctions include "although," "because," "if," "when," "while," "since," "unless," and "whereas." For instance:
"Because it was raining, we stayed indoors." (showing cause and effect)
"Although she studied hard, she didn't pass the exam." (expressing contrast)

Correlative Conjunctions: These are pairs of conjunctions that work together to join similar elements within a sentence. Common correlative conjunctions include "either...or," "neither...nor," "both...and," "not only...but also," "whether...or," and "not...but." For example:
"You can either study now **or** fail later." (presenting alternatives)
"Not only did he bring food, **but** he also brought drinks." (joining two related ideas)

Conjunctive Adverbs: These are adverbs that function as conjunctions to connect independent clauses. They indicate a relationship between the two clauses, such as cause and effect, contrast, or sequence. Common conjunctive adverbs include "however," "therefore," "consequently," "moreover," "nevertheless," and "furthermore."

For instance:

"She studied hard; **therefore**, she passed the exam." (indicating cause and effect)

"He wanted to go out; **however**, it was raining." (expressing contrast)

Usage of Conjunctions:

"And": This conjunction is used to connect words, phrases, or clauses that are similar or related, indicating addition or continuation. For example:

- "She likes to read **and** write."
- "He enjoys playing soccer **and** basketball."

"But": This conjunction is used to join contrasting ideas or clauses, indicating a contrast or exception. For example:

- "She wants to travel, **but** she doesn't have enough money."
- "He studied hard, **but** he still failed the exam."

"Or": This conjunction is used to present alternatives or choices, indicating an option or possibility. For example:

- "Would you like tea **or** coffee?"
- "You can go now, **or** you can wait for me."

"So": This conjunction is used to indicate a consequence or result, indicating cause and effect. For example:

-"It was raining, **so** we stayed indoors."
- "She studied hard, **so** she passed the exam."

Other conjunctions, such as "yet," "for," and "nor," have specific usage contexts, but they generally serve similar purposes of connecting different parts of a sentence to convey meaning effectively.

Rule 9: Capitalization Rules

Capitalization refers to the practice of using uppercase letters to denote the first letter of a word. This is to distinguish it as a proper noun, the first word in a sentence, or for emphasis. It is a fundamental aspect of writing conventions that helps readers identify important elements such as names, titles, and the beginning of sentences.

Here is a detailed explanation of capitalization rules:

Sentence Beginnings: The first word of every sentence should be capitalized. For example: "The quick brown fox jumps over the lazy dog."

Proper Nouns: Capitalize the first letter of names of specific people, places, organizations, and things. For example, "John Smith," "Paris," "Microsoft," and "Mount Everest.

Titles: Capitalize titles when they directly precede a person's name or when they are used as part of the name.
   - Example: "President Biden, Dr. Smith, Professor Johnson"
   - Exception: Do not capitalize titles when they follow a person's name or when they stand alone.
   - Example: "Joe Biden, the president of the United States"

Days of the Week, Months, and Holidays: Capitalize the names of days, months, and holidays.
For example: "Monday, December, Christmas"

Geographic Regions: Capitalize names of continents, countries, states, cities, streets, and landmarks.
For example, "Africa," "Canada," "New York City," and "The Rocky Mountains."

Nationalities and Languages: Capitalize the names of nationalities and languages.
   - Example: "American, English, Spanish"

Historical Events and Documents: Capitalize the names of specific historical events, documents, and periods.
For example, "The American Revolution," "The Renaissance," and "The Great Depression."

Religious Terms: Capitalize the names of religions, holy books, religious figures, and specific deities.
For example: "Christianity, Bible, Jesus Christ, Allah"

Titles of Works: Capitalize the principal words in titles of books, articles, movies, songs, and other works. Do not capitalize articles, conjunctions, or prepositions unless they are the first or last word in the title.
For example: "To Kill a Mockingbird, The Lord of the Rings"

First Word after a Colon: Capitalize the first word after a colon if it begins a complete sentence.
For example: "She had one hobby: Painting."

Acronyms and Initialisms:
Capitalize all letters in acronyms and initialisms, regardless of whether they form real words. For example, "NASA" (National Aeronautics and Space Administration) and "UNICEF" (United Nations International Children's Emergency Fund).

Brand Names and Trademarks:
Capitalize brand names and trademarks to distinguish them from common nouns. For example, "Coca-Cola," "Nike," and "iPhone.

Emphasis or Attention: Sometimes, words are capitalized to draw attention or indicate emphasis. However, this should be used sparingly in formal writing.
For example: "WARNING: Do Not Enter"

Rule 10: Punctuation Marks (Commas, Periods, Question Marks, Exclamation Marks)

Punctuation marks are symbols used in writing to clarify meaning, indicate pauses, separate elements, and structure sentences. They play a crucial role in conveying the intended tone, emphasis, and structure of written language. Punctuation marks include symbols such as commas (`,`), periods (`.`), question marks (`?`), exclamation marks (`!`), and many more. Each punctuation mark serves a specific purpose in guiding readers through a text and ensuring clarity and coherence in written communication.

Let's delve into these four punctuation mark in detail:

Commas (,)
 Usage:

List Separation: Commas are used to separate items in a list to make the text clearer and easier to understand. For example, "I bought apples, oranges, and bananas."
Introductory Phrases and Clauses: Commas are used to set off introductory phrases or clauses from the main part of the sentence. This helps to provide additional information or context before presenting the main idea. For example, "After finishing his homework, John went to bed."
Pauses: Commas are used to indicate pauses in sentences, helping to control the rhythm and flow of the writing. They can be used to create a natural cadence and emphasize certain parts of the sentence. For example, "The weather, however, remained unpredictable."
Clarifying Meaning: Commas are used to clarify meaning and avoid ambiguity in sentences. They can change the interpretation of a sentence or prevent misreading. For example, "Let's eat, Grandma!" (inviting Grandma to eat) versus "Let's eat Grandma!" (eating Grandma).

Periods (.)
Usage:

End a Sentence: Periods are used to mark the end of a declarative sentence, indicating a complete thought or idea. They signal that the sentence has come to a full stop. For example, "She walked to the store."

Abbreviations: Periods are used in abbreviations to indicate omitted letters or parts of words. They help to shorten longer words or phrases for convenience and brevity. For example, "Dr." for Doctor, "etc." for et cetera.

Question Marks (?)
 Usage:

Direct Questions: Question marks are used at the end of direct questions to indicate that the sentence is interrogative and requires a response. They signal inquiries or requests for information. For example, "What time is the meeting?"

Indirect Questions: Question marks can also be used in indirect questions, although this usage is less common. In this context, they still signal that a question is being asked, but the sentence is not structured as a direct question. For example, "I wonder where he went?"

Exclamation Marks (!)
 Usage:

Expressing Strong Emotions: Exclamation marks are used to convey strong emotions such as excitement, surprise, joy, anger, or urgency. They add emphasis and intensity to the statement. For example, "What a beautiful day!"

Exclamatory Statements: Exclamation marks are used in exclamatory statements to express surprise, admiration, or other strong feelings. They indicate that the statement is meant to be exclaimed rather than stated neutrally. For example, "You won the competition!"

Sentence Structure

Sentence structure refers to the way in which words are organized to form coherent and meaningful sentences. It includes the arrangement of words, phrases, and clauses within a sentence, as well as the relationships between these elements. Understanding sentence structure is crucial for you to effectively communicate with your readers or listeners as it helps convey your ideas clearly and logically. Here is an in-depth exploration of sentence structure:

Subject, Predicate, and Object

Subject:

The subject is the main noun or pronoun that performs the action or is described by the predicate in a sentence. It tells us whom or what the sentence is about. The subject typically consists of a noun, pronoun, or noun phrase. It can also be singular or plural and can appear in different positions within a sentence.

For example: "John **runs** every morning." (The subject is "John.") "John" is the subject because he is the one performing the action of running.

Predicate:

The predicate is the part of the sentence that provides information about the subject. It typically includes a verb and any accompanying words that modify or complete the action or state of being expressed by the verb.

The predicate tells what the subject is doing, what condition it is in, or what is being said about it. It can be simple or complex, depending on the structure and complexity of the sentence.

For example: "John **runs** every morning." (The predicate is "runs every morning.") It describes what John does regularly.

Object:

The object is a noun, pronoun, or noun phrase that receives the action of the verb or that is affected by the action. Objects provide additional information about the action or relationship expressed in the sentence and contribute to its overall clarity and completeness.

There are different types of objects:

Direct Object: Receives the action directly from the verb.
For example: "John eats **an apple**." (The direct object is "an apple". "An apple" is the direct object because it receives the action of eating.)

Indirect Object: Receives the direct object or benefits from the action indirectly. It indicates to whom or for whom the action is done, often preceded by a preposition.
For example: "John gives **his sister** a present." (The indirect object is "his sister because she receives the present.")

Object of a Preposition:
This appears after a preposition and completes its meaning by indicating what or who is affected by the preposition.
For example: "John walks **to the park**." (The object of the preposition "to" is "the park" because it indicates where John walks.)

Types of Sentences (Simple, Compound, Complex)

Simple Sentences:
A simple sentence consists of a single independent clause, which contains a subject and a predicate. The subject is the noun or pronoun that performs the action or is described in the sentence, while the predicate includes the verb and any additional information about the subject. It expresses a complete thought and can stand alone as a sentence.
For example: "The cat sat on the mat."
In this sentence, "The cat" is the subject, and "sat on the mat" is the predicate. Simple sentences are concise and straightforward, making them effective for conveying clear and direct statements.

Compound Sentences:

A compound sentence contains two or more independent clauses joined by coordinating conjunctions (such as "and," "but," or "or") or by semicolons (;). These independent clauses can stand alone as complete sentences. Compound sentences allow for the combination of related ideas or actions into a single sentence. They provide variety in sentence structure and can create a sense of balance or contrast between clauses.

For example: "The cat sat on the mat, and the dog played in the yard." In this compound sentence, "The cat sat on the mat" and "the dog played in the yard" are two independent clauses joined by the coordinating conjunction "and."

Complex Sentences:

A complex sentence consists of one independent clause and at least one dependent clause. A dependent clause, also known as a subordinate clause, cannot stand alone as a complete sentence because it relies on the independent clause for context and meaning. Complex sentences allow for the expression of relationships between ideas, such as cause and effect, condition and result, or other logical connections between clauses. While the dependent clause provides additional information that enhances the meaning of the independent clause.

For example: "After the cat sat on the mat, the dog barked loudly." Here, "the dog barked loudly" is the independent clause, and "After the cat sat on the mat" is the dependent clause.

In summary, simple sentences are straightforward and contain one independent clause, compound sentences combine two or more independent clauses using coordinating conjunctions or semicolons, and complex sentences include one independent clause and at least one dependent clause. Understanding these types of sentences can help writers vary their sentence structure and effectively convey their ideas.

Sentence Patterns

Sentence patterns refer to the structure or arrangement of elements within a sentence. These patterns help define how words, phrases, and clauses are organized to convey meaning. There are various sentence patterns, each with its own characteristics and purposes. Here are some common sentence patterns you should know about:

Subject-Verb (SV): This pattern forms the simplest type of sentence. It consists only of a subject and a verb. It establishes a basic relationship between the subject (the doer of the action) and the verb (the action or state). Example: "She sings." Here, "She" is the subject, and "sings" is the verb indicating the action performed by the subject.

Subject-Verb-Object (SVO): This pattern expands upon the SV pattern by adding an object, which receives the action of the verb. So it includes a subject, a verb, and an object.
Example: "He eats apples." In this sentence, "He" is the subject, "eats" is the verb, and "apples" is the object indicating what is being eaten.

Subject-Verb-Complement (SVC): In this pattern, the verb is followed by a complement that describes or renames the subject.
Example: "She is a doctor." Here, "She" is the subject, "is" is the linking verb, and "a doctor" is the complement providing additional information about the subject.

Subject-Verb-Indirect Object-Direct Object (SVOIO): This pattern involves a subject, a verb, an indirect object (recipient of the action) and a direct object (receiver of the action).
Example: "She gave him a book." Here, "She" is the subject, "gave" is the verb, "him" is the indirect object, and "a book" is the direct object.

Subject-Verb-Object-Object (SVOO): This pattern features a subject, a verb, and two objects—an indirect object followed by a direct object.
Example: "She sent him a letter." In this sentence, "She" is the subject, "sent" is the verb, "him" is the indirect object, and "a letter" is the direct object.

Subject-Verb-Adjective (SVA): This pattern is made up of a subject, a verb, and an adjective that describes the subject.
Example: "The flowers smell sweet." Here, "The flowers" is the subject, "smell" is the verb, and "sweet" is the adjective describing the subject.

Subject-Verb-Adverb (SAdv): In this pattern, an adverb modifies the verb by providing information about how, when, where, or to what extent the action is performed. Example: "She runs quickly." Here, "She" is the subject, "runs" is the verb, and "quickly" is the adverb modifying the verb "runs."

Clauses and Phrases

Clauses

A clause is a group of words that contains both a subject and a predicate (verb) and can function as a complete sentence or as part of a sentence.
For example:
"She is reading a book": In this independent clause, "She" is the subject, and "is reading a book" is the predicate, expressing a complete thought.
- "Although it was raining, we went for a walk": In this dependent clause, "Although it was raining" includes a subject ("it") and a predicate ("was raining"), but it cannot stand alone as a complete sentence. It depends on the main clause "we went for a walk" to form a complete thought.

Clauses can be independent (main clauses) or dependent (subordinate clauses).

Independent Clause: An independent clause, also known as a main clause, can stand alone as a complete sentence because it expresses a complete thought or idea. It typically contains a subject and a predicate and can function independently without being attached to another clause. For example: "She went to the store" is an independent clause because it stands alone and expresses a complete thought.

Dependent Clause: A dependent clause, also called a subordinate clause, cannot stand alone as a complete sentence because it does not express a complete thought. Instead, it relies on an independent clause to form a complete sentence. Dependent clauses often begin with subordinating conjunctions such as "although," "because," "if," "when," or "while." For instance, in the sentence "Although it was raining, we went for a walk," the clause "Although it was raining" is dependent and relies on the independent clause "we went for a walk" to form a complete sentence.

Phrases:
A phrase is a group of words that functions as a single unit within a sentence but does not contain both a subject and a predicate. Phrases can serve various grammatical purposes such as acting as nouns, verbs, adjectives, or adverbs. They provide additional information, modify other elements in the sentence, or clarify meaning within a sentence.

For example:
"The big brown dog": In this noun phrase, "the big brown" modifies the noun "dog," providing additional details about it.
"Running quickly": In this verb phrase, "running" is the main verb, and "quickly" is an adverb modifying how the action is performed.

Types of Phrases
There are four types of phrases and they include:

Noun Phrase: A noun phrase consists of a noun and any modifiers, determiners, or complements that describe or specify the noun. It functions as a noun within a sentence. These phrases function as nouns within sentences, performing roles such as subjects, objects, or complements. For example, in the phrase "the big brown dog," "the big brown" modifies the noun "dog" to provide additional information about its size and color.

Verb Phrase: A verb phrase consists of a main verb and any auxiliary (helping) verbs or modifiers that accompany it. This phrase expresses the action or state of being in a sentence. For instance, in the sentence "She is reading a book," the verb phrase "is reading" includes the main verb "reading" and the auxiliary verb "is."

Adjective Phrase: Adjective phrases function as adjectives within sentences, modifying nouns or pronouns to provide more detail or description. These phrases can include one or more adjectives along with any accompanying modifiers. For example, in the phrase "very tall and elegant," "very tall" is an adjective phrase modifying the noun "building."

Adverb Phrase: Adverb phrases function as adverbs within sentences, modifying verbs, adjectives, or other adverbs to provide information about manner, time, place, or degree. These phrases typically consist of an adverb along with any accompanying modifiers or complements. For instance, in the phrase "quite slowly and carefully," "quite slowly" is an adverb phrase modifying the verb "walked."

Active vs. Passive Voice

Active and passive voice are two different ways of constructing sentences based on the relationship between the subject and the verb. In active voice sentences, the subject performs the action expressed by the verb, while in passive voice sentences, the subject receives the action or is acted upon by the verb. Let's explain this further.

Active Voice:
In active voice sentences, the subject of the sentence performs the action described by the verb. The structure of an active voice sentence typically follows the subject-verb-object pattern, where the subject is followed by the verb and then the object (if present).

Active voice sentences are often more direct, concise, and engaging, making them preferred for most types of writing, especially when the focus is on the subject performing the action.

For example:

"The chef prepared a delicious meal for the guests." In this sentence, "the chef" (subject) performs the action of "preparing" (verb), and "a delicious meal" serves as the object of the action.

Passive Voice:

In passive voice sentences, the subject of the sentence receives the action described by the verb, rather than performing the action. The structure of a passive voice sentence often follows the object-verb-subject pattern, where the object is followed by a form of the verb "to be" (such as "is," "are," "was," or "were") and then the subject (if included).

Passive voice sentences may be useful in certain contexts, such as when the focus is on the action itself rather than the subject performing the action, or when the doer of the action is unknown or less important.

For example:

"A delicious meal was prepared for the guests by the chef." This sentence emphasizes "a delicious meal" (object) as the recipient of the action "prepared," with the agent (chef) mentioned later or left unspecified.

Key Differences Between Active and Passive Voice:

Subject Focus: Active voice emphasizes the subject performing the action, while passive voice emphasizes the action itself or the object receiving the action.

Clarity and Directness: Active voice tends to be clearer, more direct, and easier to understand than passive voice.

Verb Forms: In active voice, the verb form reflects the subject performing the action, while in passive voice, the verb form often includes a form of "to be" followed by the past participle of the main verb.

Usage: Active voice is generally preferred for most types of writing, including academic, scientific, and professional contexts, as it promotes clarity and engagement. Passive voice may be used strategically or when necessary, but should be used sparingly to avoid ambiguity or awkwardness.

Common Mistakes in Grammar

If you plan on acing the English language section of your TEAS Examination then it is important you know about the common grammar mistakes inorder to write clearly and concisely. Now, we'll look at some of the most common grammar mistakes and give their corrections.

Subject-Verb Agreement: This error occurs when the subject and verb in a sentence do not agree in number. For example, using a singular verb with a plural subject or vice versa.
Incorrect: The dogs play in the park.
Correct: The dogs play in the park.
To correct this mistake, you'll need to ensure that singular subjects are paired with singular verbs, and plural subjects are paired with plural verbs.
For example:

Misplaced or Dangling Modifiers: A misplaced modifier is a word or phrase that is positioned incorrectly in a sentence, leading to confusion or ambiguity about which word it is intended to modify. A dangling modifier occurs when the word or phrase it is intended to modify is missing from the sentence altogether.
For example:
Misplaced: Running quickly, the bus was caught by Sarah.
Dangling: Walking to the store, the rain started to fall.

To correct these errors, modifiers should be placed as close as possible to the word they modify to clarify their intended meaning.

Misuse of Verb Forms: Using incorrect verb forms, such as irregular past tense forms or incorrect verb conjugations, can lead to grammatical errors in sentences. For example, saying "He don't like ice cream" rather than "He doesn't like ice cream." This shows the use of the wrong verb tense in a sentence.

Run-On Sentences and Sentence Fragments: Run-on sentences occur when two or more independent clauses are joined without appropriate punctuation or conjunctions. This results in a sentence that lacks clarity or coherence. Sentence fragments, on the other hand, are incomplete sentences that do not contain a subject and verb or fail to express a complete thought.
For example:
Run-On: I went to the store I bought some milk.
Fragment: Without a doubt.
These errors can be corrected by separating clauses into individual sentences or by using appropriate punctuation and conjunctions to join them.

Incorrect Pronoun Usage: This mistake occurs when pronouns are used incorrectly. This leads to ambiguity or confusion about the referent they represent. Common errors include using the wrong pronoun case (e.g., "me" instead of "I"), unclear antecedents, and pronoun-antecedent agreement errors.
For example:
Incorrect: Me and him went to the movies.
Correct: He and I went to the movies.
To correct these mistakes you'll need to ensure that pronouns agree in number, gender, and case with their antecedents and that their referents are clear.

Confusion Between Homophones: Homophones are words that sound alike but have different meanings or spellings. Confusing homophones such as "there," "their," and "they're" or "its" and "it's" can lead to grammatical errors in writing.

For example:

Confused: Their going to the beach.

Correct: They're going to the beach.

To avoid these mistakes while writing, you should pay close attention to the meanings and spellings of homophones and use them appropriately in context.

Incorrect Apostrophe Usage: Misuse of apostrophes can lead to errors in grammar, particularly in relation to possessives and contractions. For example, confusing "its" (possessive form) with "it's" (contraction of "it is") or using apostrophes in plural nouns where they are not needed.

Here's another example:

Incorrect: The cat's are sleeping.

Correct: The cats are sleeping.

Confusion Between Adjectives and Adverbs: Adjectives describe nouns or pronouns, while adverbs modify verbs, adjectives, or other adverbs. Confusing the two can lead to grammatical errors in sentences. For example, using an adjective instead of an adverb to modify a verb (e.g., "He drives real slow" instead of "He drives really slowly") or vice versa.

Spelling and Punctuation: Strategies to Enhance Accuracy in Your Use Of English language.

Spelling and punctuation are crucial aspects of English language proficiency because they ensure clarity, coherence, and professionalism in writing. Here are some strategies to enhance accuracy in these areas.

Strategies for Spelling Accuracy

Spelling Rules and Patterns:

Silent Letters: You need to study to understand when certain letters are silent in words. For example, the "k" in "knee" or the "h" in "ghost."
Knowing more about these silent letters will help you spell any word correctly.

Vowel Combinations: Take the next step to learn common vowel combinations and how they are pronounced. For instance, "ea" can make different sounds in words like "eat" and "great."

Consonant Blends: This is where two or more consonants appear together but retain their individual sounds. Learning this is one great strategy to never miss words with consonant blends.
Examples of this include "bl" in "blend" and "str" in "street."

Syllable Division: Learning how to divide words into syllables will help you spell correctly as you'll be able to spell them bit by bit and how it has been pronounced. To do this, you'll need to learn to practice recognizing syllable patterns and dividing words accordingly.

Suffixes and Prefixes: Understand how adding suffixes (word endings) and prefixes (word beginnings) can change the spelling of base words. Learn the rules for adding these affixes and how they affect spelling. You can start by making a research on different suffixes and prefixes.

Tips for Remembering Spelling

Mnemonic Devices: Create mnemonic devices or memory aids that will help you remember tricky spellings. For example, "dessert" has two "s" because you always want more dessert! You can also create acronyms, rhymes, or visual images that cab help you recall the correct spelling of challenging words.

Chunking: Break longer words down into smaller, more manageable chunks or syllables. You can do this by practicing spelling each part separately before putting them together.

Personal Spelling List: Keep a personal list of words you commonly misspell or find challenging. You can also focus on words that you frequently encounter in your writing or struggle to spell correctly. Review this list regularly and practice spelling these words until you become familiar with them.

Spelling Games and Activities: Engage in spelling games, puzzles, or online activities to make learning spelling more fun and interactive. There are many apps and websites thar offer spelling games tailored to different age groups and skill levels. Use them.

Proofreading: When writing, proofread your work carefully and pay attention to spelling errors. Use spelling dictionaries, autocorrect features, or online tools to check the spelling of words you're unsure about.

Contextual Practice: You should practice spelling words in context by using them in sentences or writing paragraphs. This helps reinforce correct spelling and demonstrates how words are used in real-life situations.

By applying these strategies consistently, you can improve your spelling accuracy and become more confident in your writing. Remember that practice and patience are key to mastering spelling skills.

Proper Use of Punctuation Marks

Punctuation marks play a crucial role in conveying meaning, structure, and clarity in written communication. Here's a closer look at some common punctuation marks and how to use them:

Period (.): The period is used to indicate the end of a sentence that is a statement or a command. It is also used in abbreviations. For example:
Statement: "She went to the store."
Command: "Please close the door."
Abbreviation: "Dr. Smith will see you now."

Comma (,): Commas serve various purposes in writing:
Separating items in a list: "I like apples, bananas, and oranges."
Setting off introductory words or phrases: "In the morning, I enjoy a cup of coffee."
Separating independent clauses joined by coordinating conjunctions (and, but, or, so, etc.): "She loves to read, and he enjoys playing sports."
Setting off non-essential information (appositives, parenthetical expressions, etc.): "My brother, a talented musician, plays the guitar."

Apostrophe ('): Apostrophes have two main uses:
For indicating possession: "Sarah's book" (the book belonging to Sarah).
For forming contractions: "it's" (contraction of "it is"), "can't" (contraction of "cannot").

Colon (:): Colons are used to introduce lists, explanations, or quotations. They can also be used to indicate time in certain contexts. For example:
Introducing a list: "Please bring the following items: milk, eggs, and bread."
 Introducing an explanation or elaboration: "There's only one thing left to do: finish the project."
Introducing a quotation: "The famous line from the movie is: 'Here's looking at you, kid.'"

Semicolon (;): Semicolons are used to connect closely related independent clauses or to separate items in a list when the items contain commas. For example:
Connecting independent clauses: "She finished her work; then, she went home."
Separating items in a list with internal commas: "The team members include John Smith, CEO; Mary Johnson, CFO; and David Lee, CTO."

Question Mark (?): The question mark is used at the end of direct questions. For example:
"What time is the meeting?"
"How are you feeling today?"

Exclamation Mark (!): Exclamation marks are used to indicate strong emotion, surprise, or emphasis. For example:
"Congratulations on your promotion!"
"What a beautiful sunset!"

Guidelines for Effective Punctuation:

Clarity and Consistency: Use punctuation marks consistently and appropriately to ensure clarity in your writing. Also, avoid overusing or underusing punctuation marks, just used them appropriately.

Sentence Structure: Use punctuation marks to structure sentences effectively and convey meaning. Pay attention to your placement of commas, periods, and other punctuation marks to ensure that your sentences are grammatically correct and easy to understand.

Reading Aloud: Read what you've written aloud to check for natural pauses and breaks where punctuation marks should be placed. This will help you identify areas where punctuation is needed or where it may be misused.

Proofreading: Take the time to proofread your writing carefully for punctuation errors. Look for missing or misplaced punctuation marks, and make any necessary corrections to ensure that your writing is polished and professional.

Consistency in Style: If you're writing for a specific style guide or publication, ensure you adhere to their guidelines for punctuation usage. This is because different style guides may have slightly different rules for punctuation. So it's important to be consistent within the context of your writing.

By following these guidelines for effective punctuation, you can enhance the clarity, coherence, and professionalism of your writing, especially when answering your TEAS 7 examination questions. Remember To Practice These Before The Exam!

CONTACT THE AUTHOR

I always strive to make this guide as comprehensive and helpful as possible, but there's always room for improvement. If you have any questions, suggestions, or feedback, I would love to hear from you. Hearing your thoughts helps me understand what works, what doesn't, and what could be made better in future editions.

To make it easier for you to reach out, I have set up a dedicated email address:

epicinkpublishing@gmail.com

Feel free to email me for:

- Clarifications on any topics covered in this book
- Suggestions for additional topics or improvements
- Feedback on your experience with the book
- Any problem (You can't get the bonuses for example, please before releasing a negative review, contact me)

Your input is invaluable.

I read every email and will do my best to respond in a timely manner.

GET YOUR BONUSES

Dear reader,

First and foremost, thank you for purchasing my book! Your support means the world to me, and I hope you find the information within valuable and helpful in your journey.

As a token of my appreciation, I have included some exclusive bonuses that will greatly benefit you.

To access these bonuses, scan the QR Code with your phone:

Once again, thank you for your support, and I wish you the best of luck in your Exam. I believe these bonuses will provide you with the tools and knowledge to excel.

Made in United States
Troutdale, OR
03/30/2024

18848840R00133